For Sophia.
Cooking with and for you is
one of my life's greatest joys.
I love being your mom,
and I hope you'll make
some of these recipes
for me one day.

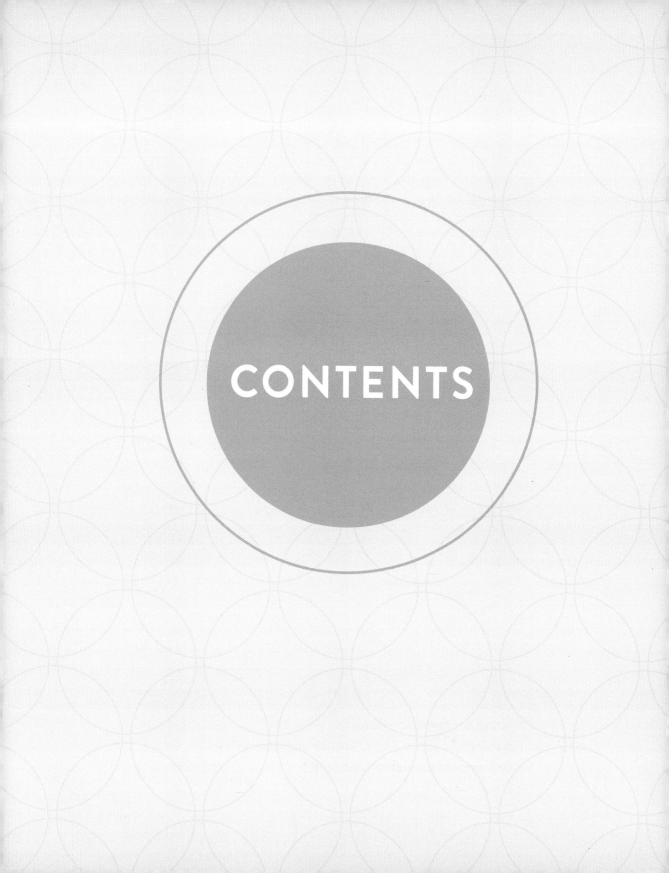

CONTENTS

Lose Weight by Eating
EASY DINNERS

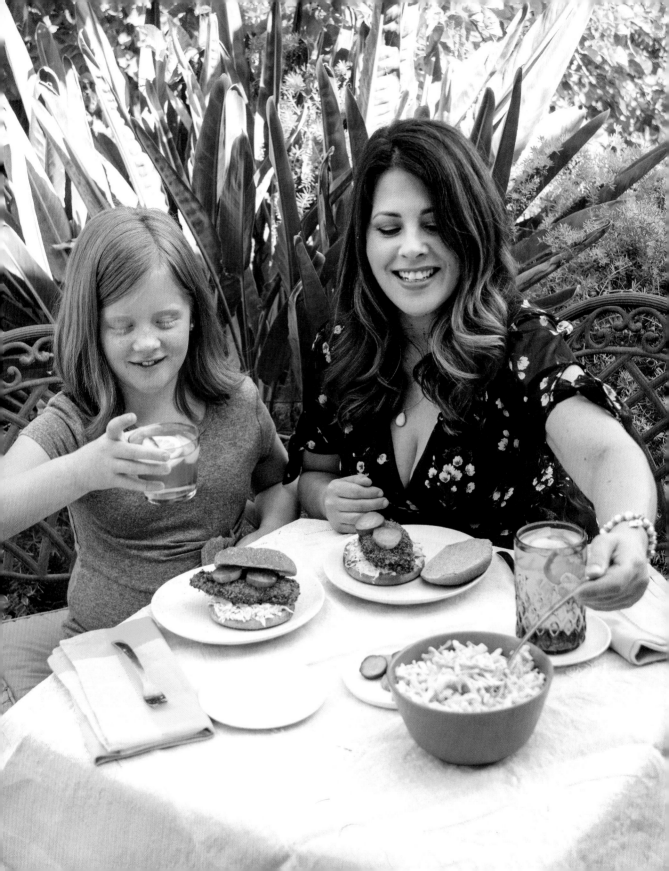

Lose Weight by Eating
EASY DINNERS

Weight Loss Made Simple with
60 Family-Friendly Meals Under 500 Calories

AUDREY JOHNS

WILLIAM MORROW
An Imprint of HarperCollins*Publishers*

Also by Audrey Johns

Lose Weight by Eating: 130 Amazing Clean-Eating Recipe Makeovers for Guilt-Free Comfort Food

Lose Weight by Eating: Detox Week

Lose Weight with Your Instant Pot

FIRST EDITION

Designed by Michelle Crowe

Circle pattern by Tongthan/ Shutterstock, Inc.

Library of Congress Cataloging-in-Publication Data has been applied for.

ISBN 978-0-06-297471-6

20 21 22 23 24   LSC   10 9 8 7 6 5 4 3 2 1

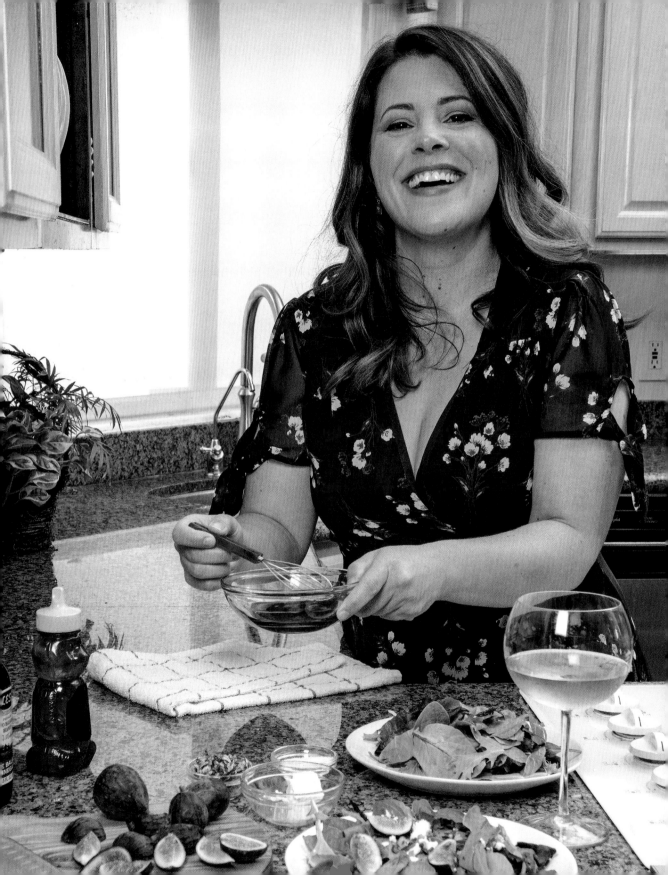

INTRODUCTION

When my editor and I started talking about a "dinner" cookbook, we didn't quite realize what it would morph into. It started out as a simple cookbook filled with recipes to answer the nightly question, "What's for dinner?" and quickly morphed to focus on the primary need for today's busy families: *easy* dinners.

To define "easy," we came up with four guidelines. Every recipe should fall into at least two of these categories to ensure the recipes were simple and easy enough for weeknight cooking:

- A recipe would take 30 minutes or less to cook.
- A recipe would take 5 minutes or less to prep.
- A recipe would contain 5 ingredients or fewer (not counting salt, pepper, olive oil, and water).
- A recipe would feature "dump everything in and walk away"-style cooking.

But more important than any guideline, I wanted the recipes to be really tasty, and I was worried that these parameters might mean less-than-delicious meals. But as I worked, I found shortcuts (like dump-and-walk-away Beef Bourguignon, page 38) and turned impressive, time-consuming meals into easy-to-make dinners. To do this, I leaned heavily on pantry staples (more on this on page 5) to cut prep or cooking times and to increase the ease of cooking.

I also wanted to be sure all the meals had under 500 calories per serving; this way you have room for dessert or a glass of wine (or a second helping, even). So, you can rest easy knowing every meal in this book will support your personal calorie budget.

Finally, I hear from readers all the time, and I wanted to take their requests and needs into account. The main request I get is for more vegetarian or vegan meals, and I'm happy to tell you that 50 percent of the recipes in this book are either meatless or include an easy meatless modification. For my vegetarian and vegan readers, I have even added a list at the back of the book so you can quickly scan the meatless meals for yourself (see page 141–42).

I'll go into more depth on this in chapter 1, but I am a firm believer that dinner is the most important meal of the day. Not for nutrition, but for its social aspect. I hope this cookbook brings your family and friends together over delicious meals. I hope it brings your kids into the kitchen to help you cook (see page 75 for tips on cooking with kids), and I hope it makes your evenings easier and more delicious.

HAPPY COOKING XO

DINNER . . . THE MOST IMPORTANT MEAL OF THE DAY

Why is dinner the most important meal of the day? It has nothing to do with dietary reasons and everything to do with the large role it plays socially.

I've been writing, coaching, and working in the weight loss world for ten years now, and in all my work I've found that dinner is most people's Achilles' heel when it comes to weight loss. It's the most social meal of the day; it's the last meal of the day; it's typically prepared at the end of a long day; and it's often the biggest meal of the day. For all these reasons, it tends to be a nightly struggle to prepare, especially when it comes to eating healthy and maintaining portion control.

Fatigue surrounding dinner is so common that companies are creating dinner boxes to deliver your meals to you weekly. These wonderful meals are unfortunately very expensive and often not prepared with health and nutrition in mind. Sure, they're less expensive than going out . . . but not by much!

We've all experienced the dinner dilemma over the years. From frozen dinners to drive-throughs, meal prep, and slow-cooking and fast-cooking meals, we've all tried ways to make dinner more accessible. Dinner may always be a challenge, but this book is meant to simply make things work better. It will help make dinner easier and more convenient, healthier and more social, less stressful and more fun.

My goal for you, as you read and cook from this book, is to have you cook more dinners each week. That can be a solo job for you, the reader, or a teaching moment for you and your children (see chapter 6 for kid-friendly meals), or a romantic moment for you and your partner (honestly, it's pretty sexy cooking with, or for, someone you love). I hope you can find a way to enjoy your dinner preparation. I hope you find that cooking with or for friends and family can be as social as going out. And—my hope of all hopes—I pray that you include your kids in the cooking process, even if they aren't actively cooking with you.

My eleven-year-old daughter, Sophia, knows so much about food. Yes, she does cook with me sometimes, but more often she sits at the kitchen island and does her homework or plays her online games while I'm making dinner. She also learns by watching, and I always want her to be part of the process. It's our job to teach our kids to cook, to teach them about food, and, most important, to teach them how to eat healthy. If not us, then who?

One of my earliest memories is of my mom encouraging me to brush my teeth. She would come to my bathroom to brush her own teeth, too. She would ooh and ahh at the smell of the toothpaste and exclaim over and over how good it felt to brush properly. Now, we all know that brushing your teeth is not as gratifying as a 60-minute massage, but she sure sold me on it. She taught me that even routine and necessary tasks could be done with joy.

What if you could show your kids that making dinner is a joyful event? Blast your favorite tunes and dance your way around the kitchen, shush everyone and tell them it's your special time—the kitchen is your sanctuary—or ask them if they want to "play" with you in the kitchen. Convince them (and yourself) that this necessary job can be done with joy. After a while you'll love your cooking time, and your kids will learn how to properly brush their teeth . . . I mean, learn to love cooking.

You can tell I'm passionate about dinner, can't you?! I am. . . . In fact, I believe family dinner, with everyone sitting around the table, is the answer to a lot of the disconnect we are seeing among family members. Of course, having those meals together every day is ideal, but what if you just made one night a week a family meal night? One night a week, you all sat around a table (without phones or devices!) and had a meal together? Sunday night is a good option since most people don't work Sundays (or if you do, choose a different day to be "your" Sunday). You can make a huge meal and save leftovers for the week to make dinner easier going forward, and it's a fantastic time to sit down and talk about your wins that week and the goals for the next.

Breakfasts are consumed in a rush, lunches are often eaten out of the home. . . . Let's take dinner back!

Planning Is Key!

A well-planned dinner will set you up for success all day long. If you know you have a delicious, healthy dinner coming up tonight, you'll be more likely to stick to your breakfast, lunch, and snack plans throughout the day.

Planning a week's worth of dinners can be very helpful for time and budget management! Of course planning your dinners will mean you don't have to visit the grocery store daily, but it's not just about limiting your trips to the store. If you plan a week's worth (or even three nights' worth) of dinners, you can better utilize your ingredients and save money!

Pantry Staples

Keeping a well-stocked pantry means you can toss dinner together in a flash. Keep in mind, Lose Weight by Eating recipes will never include preservatives, food dyes, or fake sugars. These chemically based ingredients often negatively affect weight loss, cause weight gain, and can even make you sick. So instead of buying a packet of premade ranch seasoning, flip to page 137 for a preservative-free version.

When shopping for pantry items, I recommend buying extra of any ingredients on sale. It can also be useful to keep a list on your phone of the more expensive "investment ingredients" you want to purchase. That way, whenever you shop (whether or not you're cooking with that ingredient that week), you can scout out discounts to take advantage of.

There are five major areas of your pantry to keep stocked:

- Herbs and spices
- Baking goods
- Canned and jarred foods
- Boxes of pasta and rice
- Toppings

HERBS AND SPICES

I can't tell you how often I hear from people, "Chicken is boring!" And yes, it can be . . . if you keep making the same chicken with salt and pepper and nothing else on it. Changing up your herbs and spices for each meal can keep your taste buds happy and, at zero calories, your waistline as well.

I always prefer fresh herbs, but I keep dried herbs on hand, too.

- My favorite dried herbs to have on hand are Italian seasoning, dill, cilantro, and basil.
- My favorite spices to have on hand are garlic salt or powder, chili powder, cumin, cayenne pepper, and turmeric.

BAKING GOODS

These are just the basic necessities, should you desire pancakes or pizza crust or need to bake a birthday cake.

- All-purpose flour
- Baking soda and baking powder
- Sugar (I keep raw sugar, coconut sugar, powdered, light, and dark brown sugar in my pantry)
- Rolled oats
- Chocolate chips
- Dried fruit (such as cranberries and raisins)

CANNED AND JARRED FOODS

I love that I can find BPA-free cans at my local store! I keep so many cans in my home that it's dizzying . . . but it's also inexpensive, and when I find canned foods on sale, I stock up big time.

- Cans of beans (I always keep black beans, pinto beans, and chickpeas stocked)
- Cans of crushed tomatoes and tomato paste for sauces
- Cans or cartons of chicken broth and vegetable broth
- Canned tuna
- Jars of coconut oil
- Jars of curry paste

BOXES OF PASTA AND RICE

Somewhere in this book I talk about my pasta-hoarding tendencies, and it's no joke—I have more pasta in my home than any one person should. It's a bit much, but when I find boxes of pasta on sale for $1 at the store . . . I can't help myself.

- Pasta (including spaghetti, rigatoni, and penne, both traditional and gluten-free versions)
- Rice
- Panko or other bread crumbs
- Crunchy taco shells
- Quinoa

TOPPINGS

This is the hodgepodge part of my pantry, containing toppings for everything from salad to baking. Toppings that you can store in your pantry are key; they last forever—and you can fancy up any meal if your toppings are well stocked.

- Nuts and seeds
- Unsweetened dried fruits
- Unsweetened coconut flakes
- Sun-dried tomatoes
- Sprinkles in all the colors of the rainbow

Lose Weight by Eating
GROCERY LIST

PRODUCE

CANNED AND JARRED

DAIRY

MISC.

MEAT/PROTEIN

MIX-AND-MATCH
SOUPS AND SALADS

love the combination of soup and salad for dinner. The idea for this chapter is to pick a soup and a salad and combine them into one fantastic meal. Of course, you could serve one as a side dish, or get fancy and serve one as a first course to an entrée from a later chapter.

My favorite combinations are the Sweet Pumpkin Squash Soup and Simple Greek Salad (*cough* Panera) and the Broccoli-Cheese Soup and BLTA Salad (sprinkle a few extra crumbles of the bacon from the salad onto the soup . . . heaven!).

Miso Soup

Did you know that most restaurants serve miso soup that contains gluten? Of course, if you're not gluten sensitive, that's not important . . . but when you're dating someone who is both gluten intolerant and loves miso soup, it is!

I ordered gluten-free miso paste online just for him . . . but if you don't avoid gluten, you can get traditional miso paste at the grocery store. If it's hard to find, ask for help, but usually it's in the refrigerated organic section or the Asian foods section.

◯ **SERVING SIZE:** 1 cup   **PREP TIME:** 2 minutes   **COOK TIME:** 5 minutes
PER SERVING: *calories 32; fat 1 g; saturated fat 0 g; fiber 0.5 g; protein 2 g; carbohydrates 5 g; sugar 1 g*

---

1 sheet dried nori (seaweed for sushi)
4 cups (1 quart) low-sodium vegetable broth
2 tablespoons miso paste
¼ cup diced extra-firm tofu
2 green onions, thinly sliced

1. Cut the nori in half, then slice it into thin strips. Set aside.

2. In a medium saucepan, bring the broth to a simmer over medium heat. Add the nori and cook for 5 minutes to soften it.

3. Use a coffee mug to scoop about ¼ cup of the hot broth from the pan. Add the miso paste to the broth in the mug and whisk well to dissolve it and break up any lumps, then return the contents of the mug to the pan. Add the tofu and green onions.

4. Remove from the heat, mix well, and serve hot.

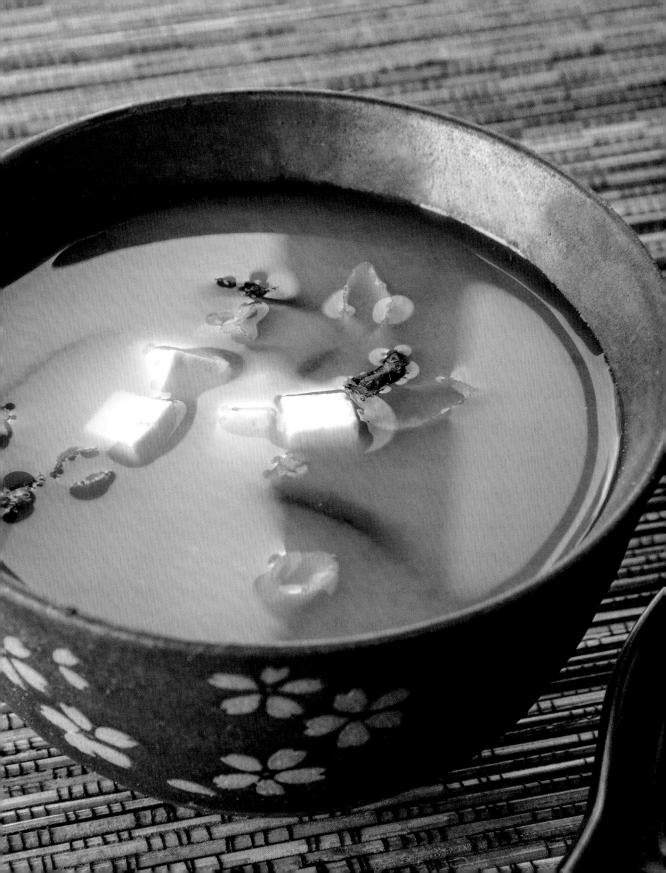

Broccoli-Cheese Soup

I love a blended soup recipe. You don't have to be precise with your chopping, so it makes for an effortless meal!

I like to pair this soup with BLTA Salad (page 23). I hold a tiny bit of the bacon back from the salad and top the soup with it. It's so delicious and doesn't add any extra calories . . . it's just a *repurposing* of calories.

You could make this dish gluten-free by using your favorite gluten-free flour mix in place of the all-purpose flour.

◯ **SERVING SIZE:** 1 cup   **PREP TIME:** 5 minutes   **COOK TIME:** 25 minutes
PER SERVING: *calories 103; fat 3 g; saturated fat 1 g; fiber 2 g; protein 11 g; carbohydrates 9 g; sugar 4.5 g*

---

1 tablespoon unsalted butter
1 medium yellow onion, roughly chopped
3 garlic cloves, roughly chopped
1 tablespoon all-purpose flour
3 cups vegetable broth
3 cups unsweetened almond milk
5 cups broccoli florets (about 2 heads)
¼ cup shredded cheddar cheese
Kosher salt and freshly ground black pepper
0% Greek yogurt

OPTIONAL TOPPINGS
Shredded cheddar cheese
Minced fresh chives
Crumbled cooked bacon or turkey bacon

1. In a large saucepan, melt the butter over medium heat. Add the onion and sauté for 5 to 10 minutes, until it starts to soften. Add the garlic and cook for 1 minute, then add the flour and whisk to combine.

2. Add ½ cup of the broth and whisk well, breaking up any lumps. Add the remaining 2½ cups broth, the almond milk, and the broccoli. Bring to a boil, then reduce the heat to low and simmer for 10 minutes, stirring occasionally, until the broccoli is soft.

3. Remove from the heat and use an immersion blender to blend the mixture into a smooth soup. Add the cheddar, taste, and season with salt and pepper. (Alternatively, let the soup cool slightly and blend in a traditional blender with the cheddar, but be sure to vent the top to avoid an explosion of hot soup.)

4. To serve, pour 1 cup of the soup into a bowl and mix in 1 tablespoon (or 2, should you love it as much as I do) of the Greek yogurt. This will thicken up the soup and add creaminess.

Butternut Squash Bisque

🍲 **MAKES 8 SERVINGS**

I am obsessed with butternut squash; it's just the prettiest color ever! This soup is the perfect fall dish. I like to pair it with Kale Caesar Salad (page 26) for a hearty and filling meal.

◯ **SERVING SIZE:** 1 cup   **PREP TIME:** 5 minutes   **COOK TIME:** 30 minutes
PER SERVING: *calories 183; fat 9 g; saturated fat 1.5 g; fiber 3.5 g; protein 8 g; carbohydrates 19 g; sugar 4.5 g*

Olive oil spray
2 large carrots, roughly chopped
1 medium yellow onion, roughly chopped
1 (2- to 3-pound) butternut squash, peeled, seeded, and cut into 1-inch chunks
Kosher salt and freshly ground black pepper
4 garlic cloves, roughly chopped
4 cups (1 quart) vegetable broth
⅛ teaspoon ground nutmeg, plus more for garnish
½ cup unsweetened almond milk
¼ cup hulled pumpkin seeds (optional)

1. Heat a large saucepan over medium heat. Lightly spray it with olive oil, then add the carrots, onion, squash, and a light sprinkle of salt and pepper. Cook for 5 minutes, stirring often to avoid burning, then add the garlic and cook for 2 minutes, stirring often.

2. Add the broth and nutmeg, cover, and bring to a boil. Reduce the heat to maintain a simmer and cook for 20 minutes, or until the squash and carrots are soft when poked with a fork. Remove from the heat, then use an immersion blender to blend the soup until smooth. (Alternatively, use a traditional blender, but be sure to vent the top to avoid an explosion of hot soup.)

3. Stir in the almond milk. Taste and adjust the salt and pepper as desired. Serve sprinkled with the pumpkin seeds, if desired, and a dash of nutmeg.

Sweet Pumpkin Squash Soup

Panera makes an amazing squash soup, so naturally I wanted to re-create it and slash the calories drastically. Now, I'm not knocking their squash soup—it's a healthy option when eating out (I get a salad with it). But if you want to make your own at home, this will save you 140 calories and 10 grams of fat per serving.

Remember, you're going to use a blender to pulverize all the ingredients, so there is no need to chop precisely. I like to chop the onions, get them cooking, and keep prepping, to save time.

⊙ **SERVING SIZE:** 1 cup   **PREP TIME:** 5 minutes   **COOK TIME:** 30 minutes
PER SERVING: *calories 103; fat 2.5 g; saturated fat 1 g; fiber 3.5 g; protein 4 g; carbohydrates 18 g; sugar 8.5 g*

1 teaspoon olive oil
1 medium yellow onion, roughly chopped
1 (1- to 2-pound) butternut squash, peeled, seeded, and cut into 1-inch chunks
3 carrots, roughly chopped
3 sweet apples (Honeycrisp and Gala are good), peeled, cored, and roughly chopped
8 cups (2 quarts) vegetable broth
1 teaspoon mild curry powder
½ teaspoon pumpkin pie spice
1 (15-ounce) can unsweetened pumpkin puree
3 ounces light cream cheese (Neufchâtel cheese)
1½ tablespoons dark or light brown sugar
Kosher salt and freshly ground black pepper

1. In a large saucepan, heat the oil over medium-low heat. Add the onion and sauté for 5 minutes, or until softened. Add the squash, carrots, apples, broth, curry powder, and pumpkin pie spice. Cover and bring to a boil. Reduce the heat to maintain a simmer and cook for 15 minutes, or until the squash is soft when poked with a fork. Stir in the pumpkin puree and remove from the heat.

2. Add the cream cheese and use an immersion blender to blend the soup until smooth. (Alternatively, use a traditional blender, but be sure to vent the top to avoid an explosion of hot soup.)

3. Season with salt and pepper to taste and serve hot.

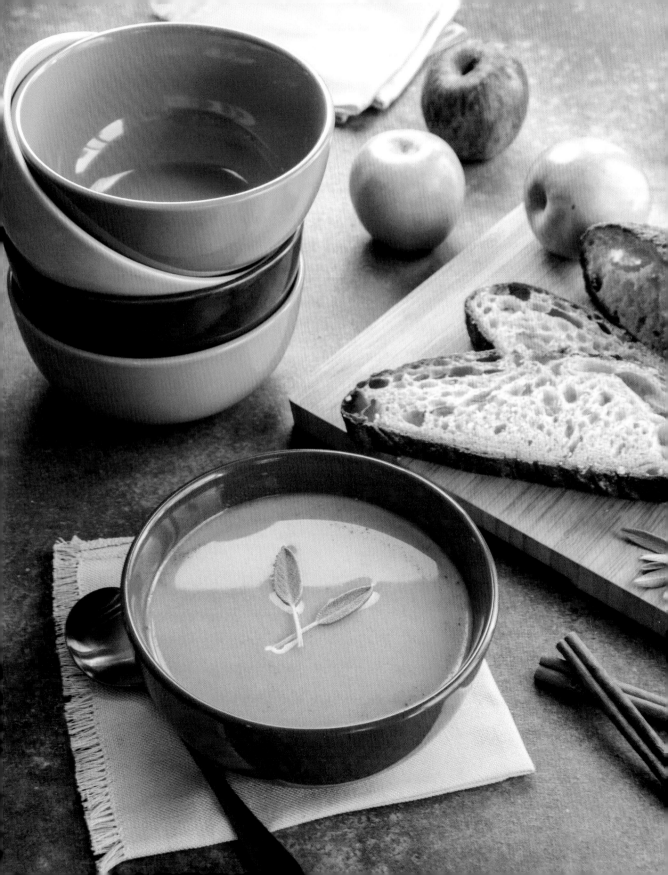

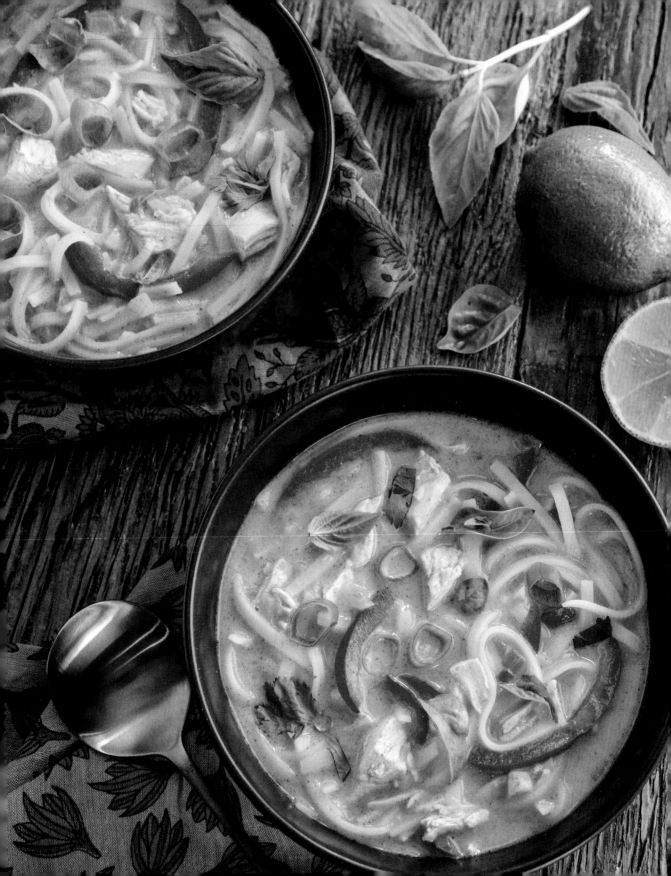

Chicken Curry Soup

🥫 **MAKES 8 SERVINGS**

I can't get enough of this soup. It's so unique and delicious! I love the subtle heat of the curry and the bite of the lime juice. If you're not crazy about curry and want to acquire a taste for it, this soup is a great introduction for your taste buds.

SERVING SIZE: 1 cup **PREP TIME:** 5 minutes **COOK TIME:** 30 minutes
PER SERVING: *calories 260; fat 16.5 g; saturated fat 11.5 g; fiber 2 g; protein 15 g; carbohydrates 12 g; sugar 3.5 g*

---

1 teaspoon olive oil
1 medium yellow onion, minced
1 red bell pepper, thinly sliced
3 garlic cloves, minced
¼ cup Thai red curry paste
6 cups (1½ quarts) chicken broth
Juice of 1 lime
1 (13.5-ounce) can light coconut milk
2 cups shredded cooked chicken
5 ounces rice noodles
Kosher salt and freshly ground black pepper
½ cup fresh basil leaves, torn
¼ cup fresh cilantro leaves, chopped
2 green onions, thinly sliced

1. In a large saucepan, heat the oil over medium heat. Add the onion and bell pepper and cook for 10 minutes, or until soft. Mix in the garlic and curry paste and cook for 1 minute.

2. Pour in the broth and lime juice and bring to a boil.

3. Add the coconut milk, chicken, and rice noodles. Cook for 10 to 15 minutes, until the noodles are al dente. Season with salt and black pepper to taste.

4. Serve hot, topped with the basil, cilantro, and green onions.

Mix-and-Match Soups and Salads

19

Chicken and Rice Soup

🍲 MAKES 8 SERVINGS

This cure-all soup will have you feeling better in no time! I added turmeric to the recipe, partially for its lovely color, but more for its cold- and flu-busting abilities!

If your nose is all stuffed up, and you can handle the heat, add a minced jalapeño to the soup when you add the red bell pepper.

SERVING SIZE: 1 cup   **PREP TIME:** 5 minutes   **COOK TIME:** 25 minutes
PER SERVING: *calories 254; fat 2.5 g; saturated fat 0.5 g; fiber 2 g; protein 13 g; carbohydrates 43 g; sugar 3 g*

1 teaspoon olive oil
2 (4-ounce) boneless, skinless chicken
  breasts, quartered
2 celery stalks, diced
3 carrots, diced
1 medium yellow onion, diced
1 red bell pepper, diced
Kosher salt and freshly ground black pepper
2 garlic cloves, minced
1 teaspoon minced fresh thyme leaves
½ teaspoon ground turmeric
½ teaspoon paprika
6 cups (1½ quarts) chicken broth
2 cups cooked white rice (I keep packaged
  cooked rice on hand for this)

1. In a large saucepan, heat the oil over medium-low heat. Add the chicken, celery, carrots, onion, and bell pepper. Sprinkle with salt and black pepper to taste and cook for 10 minutes, stirring occasionally, until the chicken is cooked through.

2. Pull the chicken out and transfer it to a plate to cool. Shred it with two forks.

3. Meanwhile, add the garlic, thyme, turmeric, and paprika to the vegetables in the saucepan. Give the spices and vegetables a quick mix, then add the broth. Bring to a boil over medium-high heat, then reduce the heat to maintain a simmer and cook for 15 minutes, or until the vegetables are soft.

4. Return the chicken to the pan and add the rice. Season with salt and black pepper to taste and serve hot.

Simple Greek Salad

🥫 **MAKES 2 SERVINGS**

This easy-to-toss-together salad is a crowd-pleaser! It's simple and elegant, and goes great with practically any meal. I like to jazz it up by adding leftover Shredded Citrus Chicken (page 90) and/or Saffron Rice (page 114).

If you don't like olives, you can swap them out for peperoncini. And if you're looking to make this a vegan recipe, swap out the feta for your favorite hard vegan cheese, or just omit the cheese altogether.

⊚ **SERVING SIZE:** 2 cups   **PREP TIME:** 5 minutes   **COOK TIME:** 0 minutes
PER SERVING: *calories 183; fat 15 g; saturated fat 4.5 g; fiber 2.5 g; protein 5 g; carbohydrates 10 g; sugar 5 g*

DRESSING
1 tablespoon extra-virgin olive oil
1 tablespoon balsamic vinegar
Juice of 1 orange
Kosher salt and freshly ground pepper

SALAD
1 large head romaine lettuce,
    cut into bite-size pieces
1 cup halved cherry tomatoes
1 cup thinly sliced cucumber
4 tablespoons crumbled feta cheese
½ cup pitted Kalamata olives

1. Make the dressing: In a mason jar or in a small bowl, combine the oil, vinegar, orange juice, and salt and pepper to taste. Cover and shake or whisk together and set aside.

2. Assemble the salad: In a large bowl, combine the romaine, tomatoes, cucumber, 2 tablespoons of the feta, and the olives. Add the dressing and toss to combine. Top with the remaining 2 tablespoons feta and dig in.

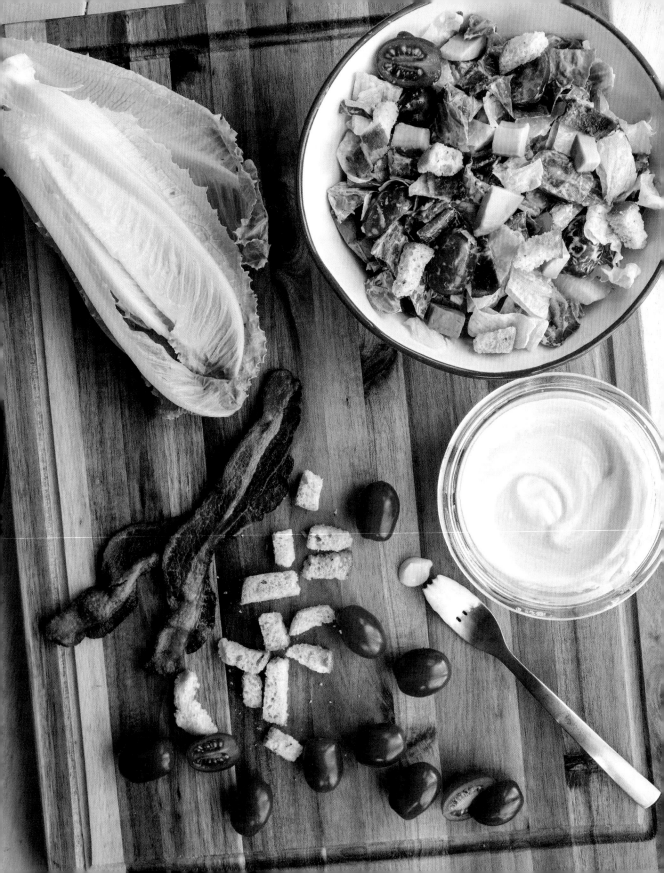

BLTA Salad

Do you know what's better than a BLT? A BLTA! And do you know what's better than a bacon, lettuce, tomato, avocado sandwich? A BLTA salad!

Here's a healthy way to enjoy the iconic sandwich. You still get the bread . . . but in the form of croutons. See, I told you this was better than a BLTA.

I can already feel the hate mail coming in for using bacon in a "diet" book, so here's the skinny: We're using just 2 slices of bacon for 4 servings, and I find that in getting others to eat healthy, we often have to make concessions for their preferred taste. Each serving gets only ½ slice of bacon, so it's just enough to get the flavor without throwing off your diet, and as I note in the recipe, you can use turkey bacon instead.

◯ **SERVING SIZE:** 2 cups   **PREP TIME:** 5 minutes   **COOK TIME:** 10 to 15 minutes
PER SERVING: *calories 394; fat 15 g; saturated fat 2.5 g; fiber 17 g; protein 22 g; carbohydrates 50 g; sugar 32 g*

DRESSING
¼ cup 0% Greek yogurt
1 teaspoon Dijon mustard
½ teaspoon garlic powder
Kosher salt and freshly ground black pepper

SALAD
2 slices bacon (or turkey bacon)
4 heads romaine lettuce, cut into bite-size
 pieces
20 grape tomatoes (about 1 cup)
1 avocado, cut into ½-inch cubes
Croutons (optional; see page 27)

1. Make the dressing: In a small bowl, combine the yogurt, mustard, garlic powder, salt and pepper to taste, and 2 tablespoons water. Mix well.

2. Prepare the salad: In a skillet, cook the bacon over medium heat to your desired crispiness. Transfer to paper towels to absorb some of the oil.

3. In a large bowl, combine the romaine, tomatoes, and dressing. Toss to combine, then top with the avocado and croutons, if desired. Crumble the bacon over the top and serve.

Spicy Caesar Salad

One of my favorite local Boise restaurants used to make this salad, and they still do . . . kind of. They took out the kale and added some cheese. Now, the cheese is lovely, and a great addition (as you can see below, I've included it), but they took away the kale. And though I know it's not everyone's favorite green, it *makes* this salad!

I missed the old version so badly that I had to re-create the recipe at home. It took several tries to reach perfection, but here it is, in all its spicy kale glory.

⊙ **SERVING SIZE:** 2 cups   **PREP TIME:** 5 minutes   **COOK TIME:** 0 minutes
PER SERVING: *calories 247; fat 12 g; saturated fat 3 g; fiber 5.5 g; protein 12 g; carbohydrates 29 g; sugar 9 g*

DRESSING

2 jalapeños, seeds and ribs removed
½ cup fresh cilantro leaves
Juice of 1 lime
2 cups 0% Greek yogurt
½ teaspoon kosher salt, plus more if needed
¼ teaspoon freshly ground black pepper, plus more if needed

SALAD

6 cups thinly sliced kale (about 1½ bunches)
2 heads romaine lettuce, cut into bite-size pieces
1 red (or other color) bell pepper, chopped
½ cup frozen corn kernels, thawed
1 avocado, cut into medium dice
½ red onion, minced
4 tablespoons crumbled Cotija cheese
¼ cup Croutons (optional; see page 27)

1. Make the dressing: In a blender, combine the jalapeños, cilantro, lime juice, yogurt, salt, pepper, and 2 tablespoons water and blend until smooth, adding more water to thin the dressing as needed. Taste and season with more salt and pepper if needed.

2. Assemble the salad: In a large bowl, combine the kale, romaine, bell pepper, corn, half the avocado, the red onion, and 2 tablespoons of the Cotija. Add the dressing and toss to combine.

3. Top with the remaining avocado, 2 tablespoons Cotija, and the croutons (if using) and serve.

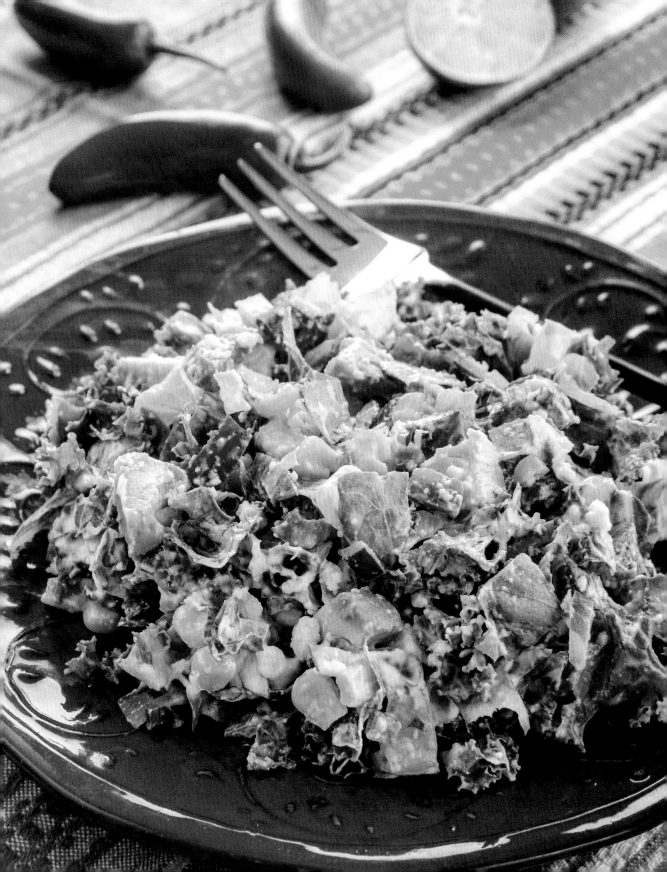

Kale Caesar Salad

I wanted to make two versions of a kale Caesar salad for this book—this one, a traditional Caesar with kale, and Spicy Caesar Salad (page 24), which is spicy with a mix of kale and romaine. Of course, if you're concerned with the "kale" aspect, you could make this half kale and half romaine as well, but I think you'll find this yummy version to be a great way to eat your leafy greens.

◯ **SERVING SIZE:** 2 cups   **PREP TIME:** 5 minutes   **COOK TIME:** 0 minutes
PER SERVING: *calories 233; fat 1 g; saturated fat 0.5 g; fiber 2 g; protein 32 g; carbohydrates 25 g; sugar 11 g*

DRESSING
⅓ cup 0% Greek yogurt
1½ tablespoons fresh lemon juice
1 teaspoon Dijon mustard
½ teaspoon garlic powder
⅛ teaspoon freshly ground black pepper

SALAD
4 cups chopped kale (about 1 bunch)
2 tablespoons freshly grated Parmesan cheese
¼ cup Croutons (optional; see page 27)
1 avocado, sliced (optional)

1. Make the dressing: In a mason jar or a small bowl, combine the yogurt, lemon juice, mustard, garlic powder, and pepper, adding water 1 teaspoon at a time until the dressing reaches your desired thickness. Cover and shake, or whisk, to combine and set aside.

2. Assemble the salad: In a large bowl, combine the kale and 1 tablespoon of the Parmesan. Top with the dressing and toss to combine. Sprinkle the remaining 1 tablespoon Parmesan on top. If desired, add the croutons and avocado, and serve.

Croutons

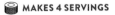

SERVING SIZE: ¼ cup   PREP TIME: 2 minutes   COOK TIME: 10 minutes
PER SERVING: *calories 33; fat 1.5 g; saturated fat 0 g; fiber 0 g; protein 1 g; carbohydrates 5 g; sugar 0 g*

1 slice of bread (I like sourdough or gluten-
   free), cut into small cubes
Olive oil spray
Kosher salt and freshly ground black pepper

1. Preheat the oven to 350°F. (If you have a toaster oven, you can toast the croutons there instead.)

2. Spread the bread cubes on a baking sheet and spray them lightly with olive oil. Sprinkle a little salt and pepper over the bread.

3. Bake for 10 minutes, or until slightly crispy (they will crisp up more as they cool). (To use the toaster oven, toast as you would a slice of bread.)

4. Let cool before serving. You can store leftovers in a sealed container for up to 1 week at room temperature.

Figs in Field Greens

This vegetarian salad makes the perfect summer meal. You know those summer evenings when it's too hot to cook? That's when figs are in season, and it's the perfect time to make this salad.

⭕ **SERVING SIZE:** 2 cups **PREP TIME:** 2 minutes **COOK TIME:** 0 minutes
PER SERVING: *calories 361; fat 22 g; saturated fat 3 g; fiber 11 g; protein 8 g; carbohydrates 39 g; sugar 24 g*

---

1 tablespoon balsamic vinegar
1 teaspoon honey
4 cups mixed greens (about a 5-ounce package)
4 fresh figs, quartered
2 tablespoons chopped pecans
1 tablespoon crumbled goat cheese

1. In a small bowl, combine the vinegar and honey and mix well.

2. Divide the greens between two plates and top with the figs, pecans, and goat cheese. Drizzle the balsamic dressing over the salads and serve.

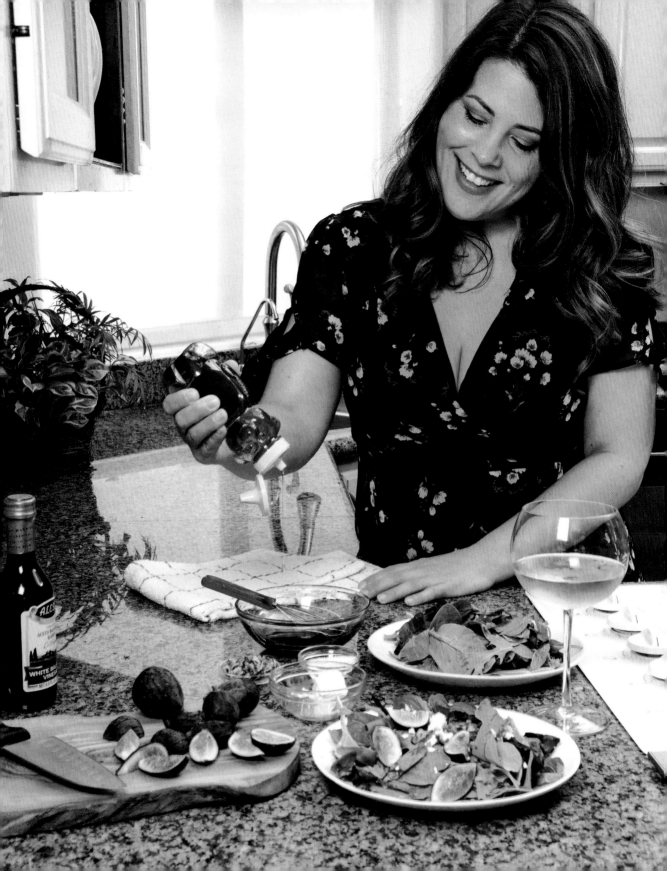

COOKING FAST/
COOKING SLOW

'm very pleased to tell you that everything in this chapter can be made in a slow cooker or an Instant Pot! Using these appliances means these recipes fall into the "easy" guidelines of this book (see page 1). Each recipe has instructions for both the fast method and the slow method, so you can choose.

Chicken Pesto Gnocchi

🥘 MAKES 4 SERVINGS

Often when I'm creating new recipes and testing them, I'll make two or three meals at once and then save them as leftovers for the end of the week when I'm busy typing up the successful recipes. Well, that backfired on this one! It was made in the Instant Pot, so it was completed before the other two meals were done, and I just . . . couldn't . . . stop . . . eating it! I was stuffed when it came time to taste-test the other recipes.

◎ **SERVING SIZE:** 1 piece of chicken and ½ cup gnocchi   **PREP TIME:** 2 minutes   **COOK TIME:** 20 minutes
PER SERVING: *calories 263; fat 3 g; saturated fat 1 g; fiber 0 g; protein 13 g; carbohydrates 46 g; sugar 0 g*

1 cup fresh basil leaves
1 teaspoon extra-virgin or regular olive oil
1 tablespoon freshly grated Parmesan cheese
2 garlic cloves
1 (16-ounce) package fresh gnocchi
4 (4-ounce) boneless, skinless chicken breasts

1. In a blender, combine the basil, oil, Parmesan, and garlic and blend until it's as smooth as you can get it. (Yes, I'm very precise.)

2. Put the gnocchi and 1 cup water in the Instant Pot. Add the trivet (the one that comes with the Instant Pot) to the inner pot and place the chicken on top. Spoon the pesto over the chicken.

3. Cover the Instant Pot and cook on high pressure for 10 minutes. Let the pressure release naturally.

4. Scoop ½ cup of the gnocchi onto each plate, top with a piece of the chicken, and serve hot.

SLOW COOKER INSTRUCTIONS

Make the pesto. Combine the chicken and ¼ cup water in the slow cooker and top with the pesto. Cover and cook on low for 3 hours. In a separate pot, cook the gnocchi according to the package directions. Serve as directed.

Tuscan Chicken and Orzo

🍥 **MAKES 4 SERVINGS**

I really love sun-dried tomatoes; they add so much flavor without adding too many calories. I recommend getting the bagged, dried version over the ones packed in oil. They're lower in calories and will last longer in your pantry.

You can make this a gluten-free dish by swapping in rice for the orzo.

○ **SERVING SIZE:** 1 cup **PREP TIME:** 3 minutes **COOK TIME:** 10 minutes
PER SERVING: *calories 325; fat 6.5 g; saturated fat 1 g; fiber 1.5 g; protein 57 g; carbohydrates 10 g; sugar 1.5 g*

2 (4-ounce) boneless, skinless
  chicken breasts
Kosher salt and freshly ground
  black pepper
½ cup orzo pasta
1 medium yellow onion, minced
½ cup unsweetened almond milk
  (or whatever unsweetened milk you
  have on hand)
½ cup chicken broth
1 teaspoon Italian seasoning
1 teaspoon garlic powder
1 cup chopped fresh spinach
¼ cup sun-dried tomatoes
2 tablespoons freshly grated Parmesan
  cheese

1. Place the chicken in the Instant Pot and sprinkle with salt and pepper. Add the orzo, onion, almond milk, broth, Italian seasoning, garlic powder, spinach, and sun-dried tomatoes.

2. Cover the Instant Pot and cook on high pressure for 10 minutes. Quick-release the pressure. Remove the chicken to a cutting board. Let sit for 5 minutes, then cut the chicken into ¼-inch-thick slices.

3. While the chicken is sitting, stir the orzo in the Instant Pot with the other ingredients and divide it among four plates.

4. Top with the sliced chicken and the Parmesan and serve.

SLOW COOKER INSTRUCTIONS

Cook on high for 2 hours or low for 3 to 4 hours.

White Chicken Chili

I love that this meal can be tossed together in a flash, and I really love that most of the ingredients are pantry and freezer staples in my home.

A well-stocked pantry (cans of beans, spices, and broth) can save you on a hectic night. Don't already have a well-stocked pantry? Make a list of all the spices and foods you want to keep in your pantry, and every time you go to the store, pick up one or two items, ideally when they are on sale!

SERVING SIZE: 1 cup   **PREP TIME:** 5 minutes   **COOK TIME:** 3 to 5 hours
PER SERVING: *calories 310; fat 3.5 g; saturated fat 1 g; fiber 10 g; protein 30 g; carbohydrates 41 g; sugar 2.5 g*

1 medium yellow or red onion, minced
1 jalapeño, seeds and ribs removed, minced
2 garlic cloves, minced
¼ cup canned diced mild green chiles
1 tablespoon ground cumin
1½ teaspoons ground coriander
1½ teaspoons chili powder
Juice of 1 lime
4 cups (1 quart) low-sodium chicken broth
2 (4-ounce) boneless, skinless chicken breasts
1 (15.5-ounce) can white beans, drained and rinsed
⅓ cup chopped fresh cilantro

OPTIONAL TOPPINGS
Shredded cheddar cheese
0% Greek yogurt (in place of sour cream)
Sliced green onions
Tortilla chips

1. In a slow cooker, combine the onion, jalapeño, garlic, green chiles, cumin, coriander, chili powder, lime juice, broth, and chicken. Cover and cook on high for 3 hours or on low for 5 hours.

2. When the chicken is almost done, put the beans in a medium bowl and use a fork to gently mash a little more than half of them. Set aside.

3. Remove the chicken breasts and shred them. Return the chicken to the slow cooker, add the beans (mashed and unmashed) and cook, uncovered, for 10 minutes to heat everything through.

4. Top with the cilantro and serve with toppings of your choosing.

INSTANT POT INSTRUCTIONS

Sauté the onion, jalapeño, garlic, green chiles, and chicken on medium in the Instant Pot, add the broth, and scrape very well so you don't get a "burn" message. Add the remaining ingredients (except the cilantro). Cover the Instant Pot and cook on high pressure for 20 minutes. Quick-release the pressure, remove the chicken and shred it, then return it to the pot and add the beans. Sauté on low for 5 minutes.

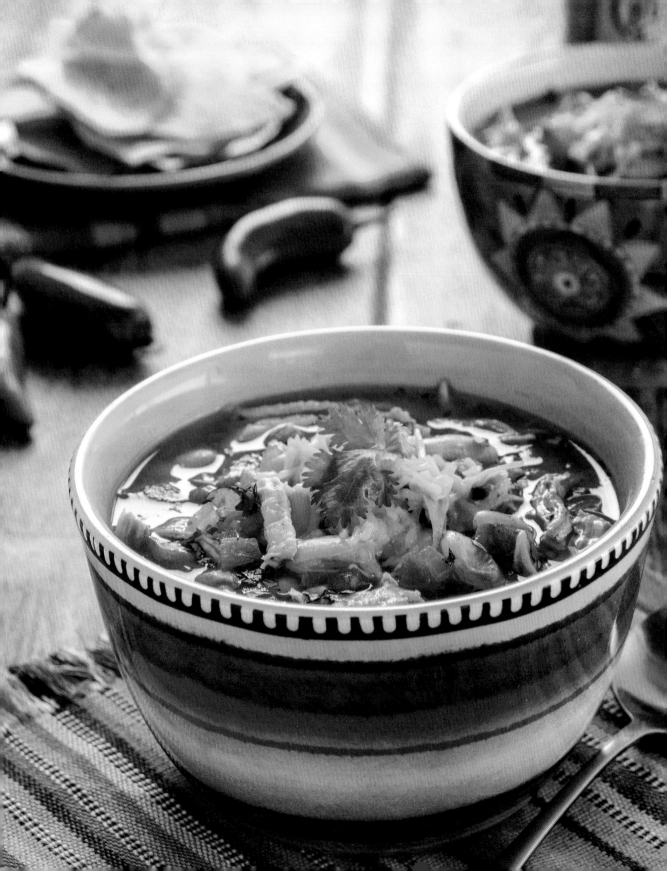

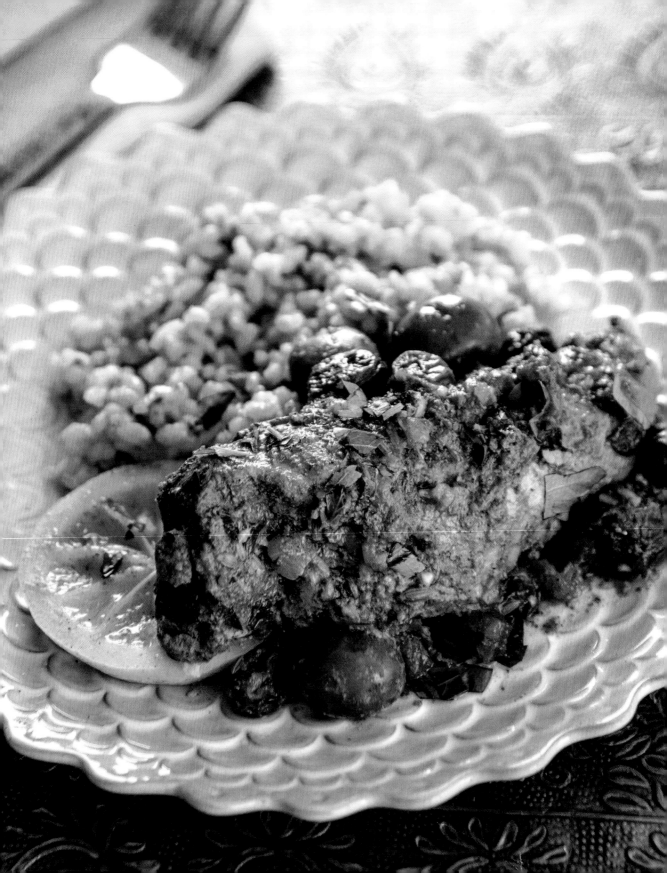

Moroccan Chicken

🥫 **MAKES 4 SERVINGS**

Wow . . . just *wow*! After I made this for the first time, I found myself mindlessly walking back to the fridge to take bites of it! It's fantastic!! And don't let the raisin and olives throw you off—this is a perfect dish.

◯ **SERVING SIZE:** 1 chicken breast   **PREP TIME:** 2 minutes   **COOK TIME:** 2 hours 30 minutes to 5 hours
PER SERVING: *calories 259; fat 7.5 g; saturated fat 1 g; fiber 2 g; protein 23 g; carbohydrates 23 g; sugar 13 g*

2 teaspoons ground coriander
2 teaspoons ground cumin
2 teaspoons ground ginger
2 teaspoons paprika
2 teaspoons ground turmeric
1 teaspoon ground allspice
1 teaspoon ground cinnamon
½ teaspoon fennel seeds
¼ teaspoon ground nutmeg
2 teaspoons chopped fresh flat-leaf parsley
¼ teaspoon kosher salt
¼ teaspoon freshly ground black pepper
2 medium red onions, roughly chopped
4 (4-ounce) boneless, skinless chicken breasts
6 garlic cloves, minced
1 cup pitted green olives
½ cup raisins
1 lemon, sliced into thick rounds

1. In a medium bowl, combine the coriander, cumin, ginger, paprika, turmeric, allspice, cinnamon, fennel seeds, nutmeg, parsley, salt, and pepper.

2. In a slow cooker, combine the onions, chicken, garlic, olives, raisins, lemon rounds, and spice mixture.

3. Mix together, cover, and cook on high for 2 hours 30 minutes or on low for 5 hours. Before serving, mix everything together to evenly disperse the spices again. Serve hot.

INSTANT POT INSTRUCTIONS

Combine all the ingredients in an Instant Pot with 1 cup water. Cover the Instant Pot and cook on high pressure for 10 minutes. Quick-release the pressure, stir to combine, and serve.

Beef Bourguignon

🥘 **MAKES 4 SERVINGS**

Since this book is all about easy dinners, I wanted to turn a classic French dish into an easy dump-and-walk-away, minimal-prep meal. This will take some strategic shopping, but these moves will not only save you time in the kitchen, they'll save you money as well.

◎ **SERVING SIZE:** 1½ cups   **PREP TIME:** 5 minutes   **COOK TIME:** 3 to 8 hours
PER SERVING: *calories 335; fat 16 g; saturated fat 6.5 g; fiber 3.5 g; protein 20 g; carbohydrates 16 g; sugar 7 g*

1 pound cubed beef stew meat, cut into bite-size pieces
2 medium onions, roughly chopped
2 cups frozen sliced carrots (no need to thaw)
2 celery stalks, sliced into 1-inch chunks
1 cup sliced white or brown mushrooms
½ cup frozen pearl onions (no need to thaw)
2 garlic cloves, minced
1 cup low-sodium beef broth
1 cup dry red wine (or more beef broth)
1 tablespoon tomato paste
2 fresh thyme sprigs, or 1 teaspoon dried thyme

1. In a slow cooker, combine the beef, onions, carrots, celery, mushrooms, pearl onions, garlic, broth, wine, and tomato paste. Give it a quick mix and place the thyme sprigs on top.

2. Cover and cook on high for 3 to 4 hours or on low for 6 to 8 hours (the longer, the better).

3. Uncover, stir to combine, remove the thyme sprigs, top with parsley, and serve hot.

INSTANT POT INSTRUCTIONS

Combine all the ingredients (except the parsley) in an Instant Pot. Cover the Instant Pot and cook on high pressure for 30 minutes. Let the pressure release naturally. Set the pot to sauté on low heat and cook, uncovered, for 10 minutes to burn off the alcohol in the wine (or swap the wine for more broth and skip this step).

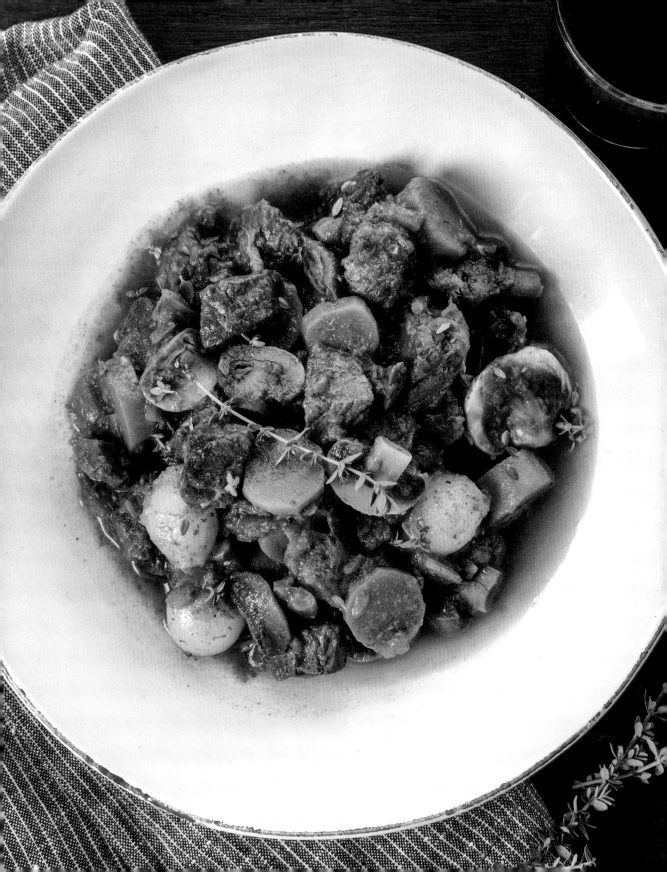

SKINNY FRIED

When I started this chapter, the idea was to supply recipes for air fryers . . . and it's still that chapter. However, I have also given directions for cooking on the stovetop or in the oven for those of you who don't have or don't want to use an air fryer.

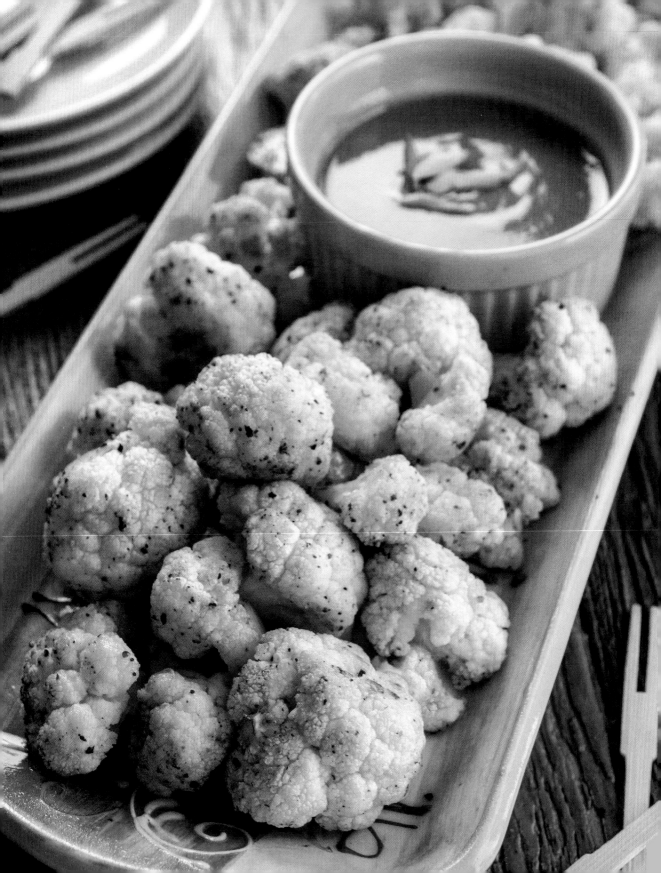

"Fried" Cauliflower Bites

MAKES 2 SERVINGS

These are a dream with or without the dipping sauce. They are crunchy and delicious and completely addictive.... You'll want to eat *all* of them in one sitting, and you can, without any guilt. That's quite a lot of food for just 106 calories!

SERVING SIZE: 2 cups   **PREP TIME:** 2 minutes   **COOK TIME:** 10 minutes
PER SERVING: *calories 53; fat 2.5 g; saturated fat 0.5 g; fiber 3.5 g; protein 3 g; carbohydrates 7 g; sugar 3 g*

1 head cauliflower, cut into bite-size florets
1 teaspoon chili powder
¼ teaspoon garlic powder
Pinch of kosher salt
Pinch of freshly ground black pepper
1 teaspoon olive oil
1 cup Buffalo Sauce (page 136) or Korean
   Barbecue Sauce (page 135)

1. Preheat an air fryer to 320°F.

2. In a large bowl, combine the cauliflower with the chili powder, garlic powder, salt, pepper, and oil and toss to coat the cauliflower in the oil and spices.

3. Place the cauliflower in the air fryer, working in batches as needed. Cook for 10 minutes, until crispy.

4. Serve with your choice of sauce on the side.

OVEN INSTRUCTIONS

Spread the coated cauliflower on a sheet pan and bake at 450°F for 15 minutes, or until crispy.

Boneless Chicken "Wings"

I made these the first time with gluten-free flour (Bob's Red Mill 1-to-1 Baking Flour) and they came out great . . . not pretty, but so tasty. And let's be honest, you're going to toss these in sauce, so they don't need to be gorgeous!

So, the moral of the story is, you can use any flour you like here, even gluten-free.

SERVING SIZE: about 10 pieces **PREP TIME:** 5 minutes **COOK TIME:** 15 minutes
PER SERVING: *calories 189; fat 2.5 g; saturated fat 0.5 g; fiber 1 g; protein 17 g; carbohydrates 24 g; sugar 0.5 g*

1 large egg
1 cup flour (all-purpose or gluten-free)
1 teaspoon chili powder
½ teaspoon paprika
¼ teaspoon cayenne pepper (optional)
¼ teaspoon kosher salt
¼ teaspoon freshly ground black pepper
2 (4-ounce) boneless, skinless chicken breasts, cut into 1-inch chunks
Olive oil spray
Buffalo Sauce (page 136), Korean Barbecue Sauce (page 135), warmed, or ranch dressing (see page 137)

1. Preheat an air fryer to 375°F.

2. In a medium bowl, whisk the egg. In a second medium bowl, combine the flour, chili powder, paprika, cayenne, salt, and black pepper.

3. Working in batches if necessary (depending on the size of your air fryer), dip the chicken in the egg, letting any excess drip back into the bowl, then dredge it in the flour mixture to coat. Spray the chicken with olive oil on all sides.

4. Place the chicken in the air fryer in a single layer with plenty of room between the pieces (do not overcrowd) and cook for 15 minutes, until crispy and cooked through with no pink in the center.

5. Use tongs to move the hot chicken to a large bowl, pour your chosen sauce over the chicken, and toss together well. Serve immediately.

OVEN INSTRUCTIONS

Dip, dredge, and spray the chicken as directed. Bake the chicken on a parchment paper–lined sheet pan at 400°F for 20 minutes.

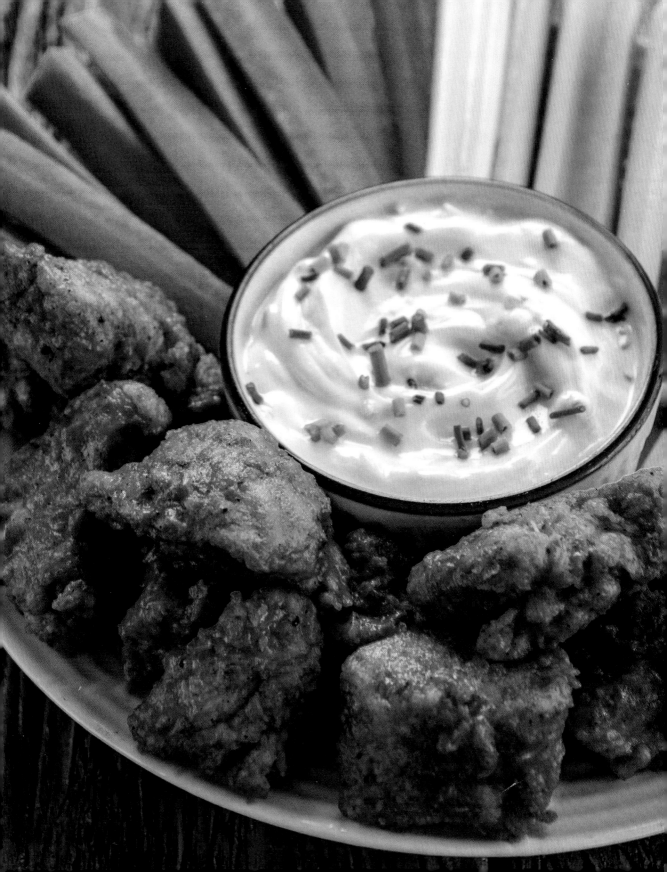

Crispy Chicken Sandwiches

🥫 **MAKES 4 SERVINGS**

These family-friendly crispy chicken sandwiches are crunchy and delicious! I love how the coleslaw adds extra crunch. If you like coleslaw, make extra and serve it as a side dish. It's healthy and easy! You can find coleslaw where you find bagged salad mix. This will save you lots of time in prepping.

⊙ **SERVING SIZE:** 1 sandwich **PREP TIME:** 5 minutes **COOK TIME:** 10 minutes
PER SERVING: *calories 357; fat 8 g; saturated fat 2 g; fiber 2.5 g; protein 32 g; carbohydrates 38 g; sugar 8.5 g*

COLESLAW
1 cup coleslaw mix
1 jalapeño, seeds and ribs removed, finely diced
¼ cup 0% Greek yogurt
½ teaspoon Louisiana-style hot sauce (I like Frank's RedHot)
¼ teaspoon garlic salt

SANDWICHES
2 (4-ounce) boneless, skinless chicken breasts
¼ cup 0% Greek yogurt
2 dashes of Lousiana hot sauce (I like Frank's RedHot)
Pinch of kosher salt
Freshly ground black pepper
½ cup panko bread crumbs (or gluten-free panko, for a gluten-free sandwich)
1 teaspoon paprika
1 teaspoon garlic salt
1 teaspoon chili powder
Olive oil spray
4 burger buns (regular or gluten-free)
8 pickle rounds

1. Preheat an air fryer to 360°F.

2. Make the coleslaw: In a medium bowl, whisk together the coleslaw mix, jalapeño, yogurt, hot sauce, and garlic salt and add water ½ tablespoon at a time until the dressing is at your desired consistency, up to 2 tablespoons. Set aside.

3. Prepare the sandwiches: Place a chicken breast on a cutting board and, using a small sharp knife, slice horizontally into the fatter side of the breast and cut all the way through to make 2 thin cutlets. (Place your hand on the top of the chicken breast as you cut through to steady it.) Repeat with the second breast.

4. Place the cutlets in a gallon freezer bag or large bowl. Add the yogurt, hot sauce, salt, a pinch of pepper, and 2 tablespoons water. Mix well and set aside in the fridge (you can do this as early as the night before).

continued

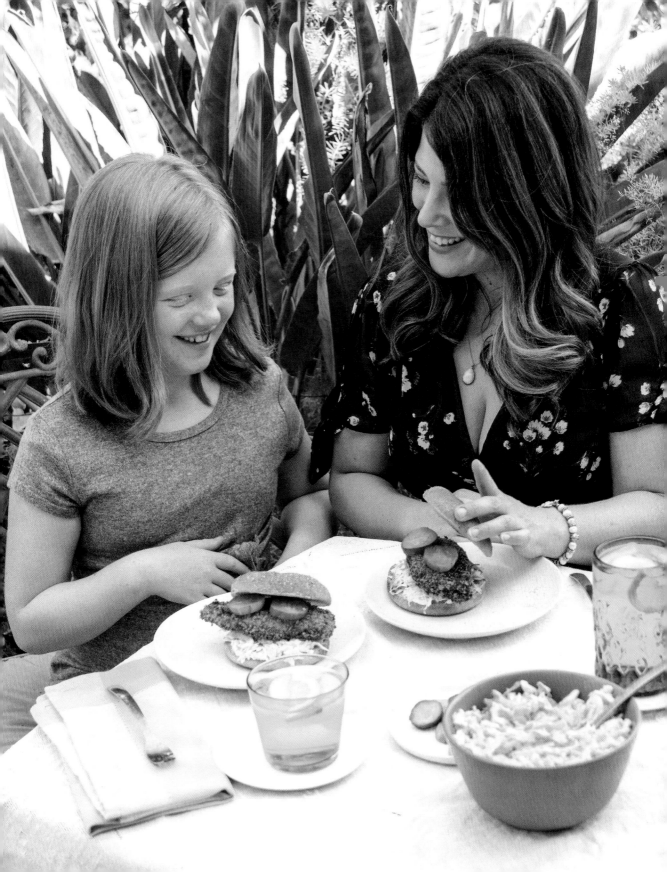

5. In a shallow bowl or pie pan, combine the panko, paprika, garlic salt, chili powder, and ¼ teaspoon black pepper. Remove a cutlet from the yogurt marinade, allowing any excess to drip off; then dredge it in the panko mixture. Spray the chicken with olive oil on all sides. Set aside on a plate and repeat to dredge the rest of the cutlets.

6. Working in batches if necessary (depending on the size of your air fryer), lay the chicken in the air fryer and cook for 10 minutes, until crispy and cooked through with no pink in the center. Use tongs to carefully remove the chicken to a plate.

7. To assemble the sandwiches, set a burger bun on each plate. Divide the coleslaw among the bottom buns and top each with a chicken cutlet, some pickles, and the top bun.

STOVETOP INSTRUCTIONS

Heat a large skillet over medium heat and cook the dredged, sprayed chicken breasts for 4 to 7 minutes on each side, until cooked through.

Chicken Schnitzel

🥫 **MAKES 4 SERVINGS**

This recipe is perhaps the lightest-tasting fried chicken I've ever had! I think it's the lemon juice that makes it taste so healthy, never too heavy. I like to make extra servings and add it to salads the next day. I just pop the chicken in the toaster oven for a few minutes and it crisps right up after a night of sitting in the fridge.

You could easily make this gluten-free by using gluten-free panko bread crumbs.

SERVING SIZE: 1 chicken cutlet   **PREP TIME:** 10 minutes   **COOK TIME:** 10 minutes
PER SERVING: *calories 199; fat 5 g; saturated fat 0.5 g; fiber 0.5 g; protein 27 g; carbohydrates 10 g; sugar 1 g*

---

1 tablespoon Dijon mustard
1 large egg
2 (4-ounce) boneless, skinless chicken breasts
½ cup panko bread crumbs
Kosher salt and freshly ground black pepper
Olive oil spray
Lemon wedges

1. Preheat an air fryer to 360°F.

2. In a shallow bowl or pie pan, whisk together the mustard and egg to combine well. Spread the panko in a second shallow bowl or pie pan.

3. Place a 3-foot piece of plastic wrap on a cutting board and lay one chicken breast in the center of the wrap. Fold the plastic wrap over so that the chicken is covered and use the flat side of a meat tenderizer (or a rolling pin) to bash it until it's flattened to ⅛ inch thick. Repeat with the second breast.

4. Lightly season both sides of the chicken cutlets with salt and pepper, then cut each piece in half to make 2 smaller cutlets (a total of 4).

5. Dip the chicken cutlets in the egg mixture, dredge them in the panko, then transfer to a plate.

6. Spray the chicken with olive oil. Working in batches if necessary (depending on the size of your air fryer), place the chicken in the air fryer and cook for 10 minutes, until crispy on the outside and cooked through with no pink in the center. Use tongs to carefully remove the chicken and plate it.

7. Squeeze lemon over each cutlet and serve with more lemon wedges.

STOVETOP INSTRUCTIONS

Dip, dredge, and spray as directed. Heat a large skillet over medium heat and cook the chicken breasts for 4 to 7 minutes on each side, until cooked through with no pink in the center.

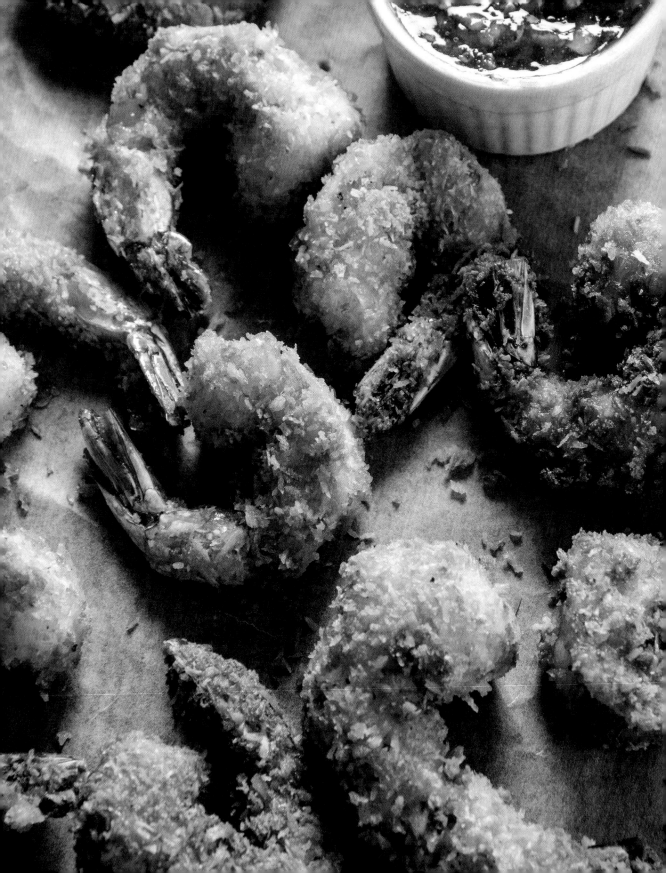

Fried Coconut Shrimp

🥫 **MAKES 4 SERVINGS**

This crunchy, flavorful dish will impress your guests—or your own taste buds, should you opt to hoard them all for yourself.

I'm allergic to shrimp, so I turned to my chef, Joni, to help me with this fantastic recipe. I'm told that she tested the recipe at the cookbook photo shoot, and seconds after the photo was done, so were the shrimp. . . . Talk about a crowd-pleaser!

Use gluten-free panko bread crumbs to make this a gluten-free meal.

◯ **SERVING SIZE:** about 8 shrimp   **PREP TIME:** 5 minutes   **COOK TIME:** 10 minutes
PER SERVING: *calories 342; fat 18 g; saturated fat 15 g; fiber 4.5 g; protein 26 g; carbohydrates 18 g; sugar 3 g*

---

1 large egg
½ cup panko bread crumbs
½ cup unsweetened shredded coconut
Pinch of kosher salt
Pinch of freshly ground black pepper
32 large shrimp, peeled and deveined
Olive oil spray

1. Preheat an air fryer to 390°F.

2. In a shallow bowl or pie pan, whisk the egg. In a second bowl or pie pan, combine the panko, coconut, salt, and pepper.

3. Working with one shrimp at a time, dip it in the egg to coat, toss it in the panko, and set it on a plate. Spray the shrimp with olive oil.

4. Working in batches if necessary (depending on the size of your air fryer), place the shrimp in a single layer with plenty of room between each one (do not overcrowd) and cook for 10 minutes, until crispy. Using tongs, remove carefully and serve.

OVEN INSTRUCTIONS

Dip, dredge, and spray as directed. Bake on a sheet pan at 425°F for 10 to 15 minutes, until crispy and cooked through.

DATE NIGHT

These date-night meals are the perfect romantic and/or impressive dish to show off your culinary talents (or to fake them!). I've made all of these for my sweetheart, but I also make the spaghetti carbonara for friends and my kiddo, so you don't have to save these recipes for date nights—any night will work.

Ginger Maple Salmon

To keep with the theme of this book, I wanted to include a five-item fish dish. It's simple and impressive and can be tossed together in minutes. If you want to spice it up a bit, serve it with Korean Barbecue Sauce (page 135) for dipping.

◎ **SERVING SIZE:** 1 portion salmon   **PREP TIME:** 5 minutes   **COOK TIME:** 20 minutes
PER SERVING: *calories 263; fat 9.5 g; saturated fat 1.5 g; fiber 1 g; protein 30 g; carbohydrates 13 g; sugar 10 g*

Grated zest and juice of 1 orange
2 teaspoons grated fresh ginger
2 garlic cloves, grated
2 tablespoons pure maple syrup
Pinch of kosher salt
Pinch of freshly ground black pepper
1 (1-pound) salmon fillet, cut into 4 portions

1. Preheat the oven to 350°F.

2. In a small bowl, combine the orange zest and juice, ginger, garlic, maple syrup, salt, and pepper. Mix the glaze well.

3. Place the salmon in a 9 × 13-inch baking dish. Spread half the glaze over the salmon.

4. Transfer to the oven and bake for 10 minutes. Spread the rest of the glaze over the salmon and bake for 10 minutes more, or until the salmon flakes when tested with a fork. Serve hot.

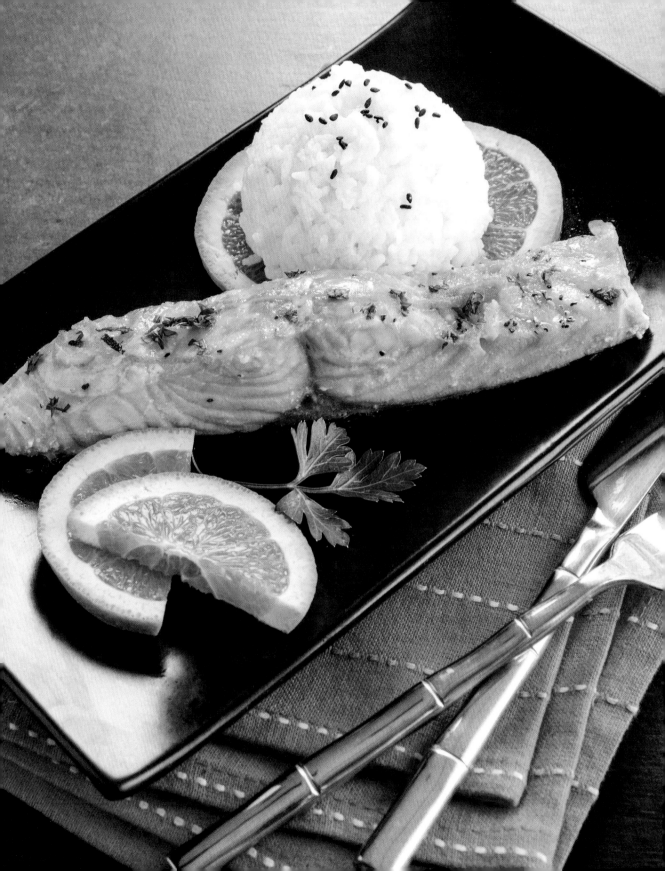

Spaghetti Carbonara

I love this pantry/freezer meal. It's impressive, and easy to toss together fast! One note: If you have a dietary concern about uncooked eggs—or if they just gross you out—simply heat the dish for 2 minutes on the lowest heat after adding the cheese.

As an Italian woman, I hoard pasta in my pantry. When I buy bacon, I freeze it in bags of 2 slices, so I always have it available—that way it never goes bad in the fridge and I don't feel obligated to eat it more often than I want to. Frozen peas always grace my freezer, and eggs, Parmesan, and garlic are always on hand in my kitchen. So when I want to make this recipe for dinner, all I might need to pick up are the kale and parsley. A well-stocked pantry lets you fulfill your romantic impulses whenever you like!

SERVING SIZE: 2 cups **PREP TIME:** 5 minutes **COOK TIME:** 25 minutes
PER SERVING: *calories 411; fat 16 g; saturated fat 7 g; fiber 8.5 g; protein 24 g; carbohydrates 47 g; sugar 2.5 g*

---

4 ounces spaghetti
1 slice bacon
1 cup thinly sliced kale
⅓ cup frozen peas (no need to thaw)
3 garlic cloves, minced
1 large egg, whisked
¼ cup freshly grated Parmesan cheese
2 tablespoons chopped fresh flat-leaf parsley

1. Bring a large pot of water to a boil. Add the spaghetti and cook until al dente according to the package directions. Before draining, reserve about ½ cup of the pasta water. (Just scoop it out with a coffee mug; it doesn't need to be precise and the mug's handle makes it safer to dip.)

2. Meanwhile, in a large skillet, cook the bacon over medium heat to your desired crispness. Crumble the bacon. Pour off all but 1 teaspoon of the bacon grease from the skillet. Return the bacon to the pan.

3. Add the kale and peas and cook for 5 minutes, stirring often, until the kale wilts and the peas thaw and warm up. Add the garlic, then remove the skillet from the heat and let cool for 3 to 5 minutes.

4. Now comes the tricky part: Add the hot pasta to the skillet, then add the beaten egg and *very* quickly mix together. If you're not quick, you'll get scrambled eggs and not sauce. If this happens, don't fret . . . just mix very well and most of the lumps will dissolve. Add ¼ cup of the reserved pasta water and mix well. Add more pasta water if needed to thin out the sauce.

5. Top with half the Parmesan and half the parsley. Toss to combine, then top with the remaining Parmesan and parsley and serve.

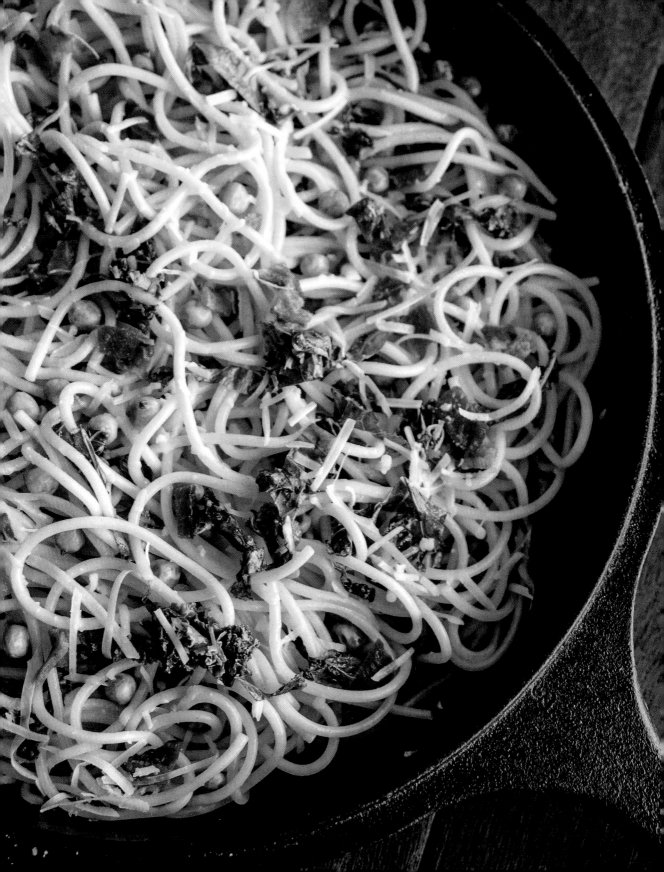

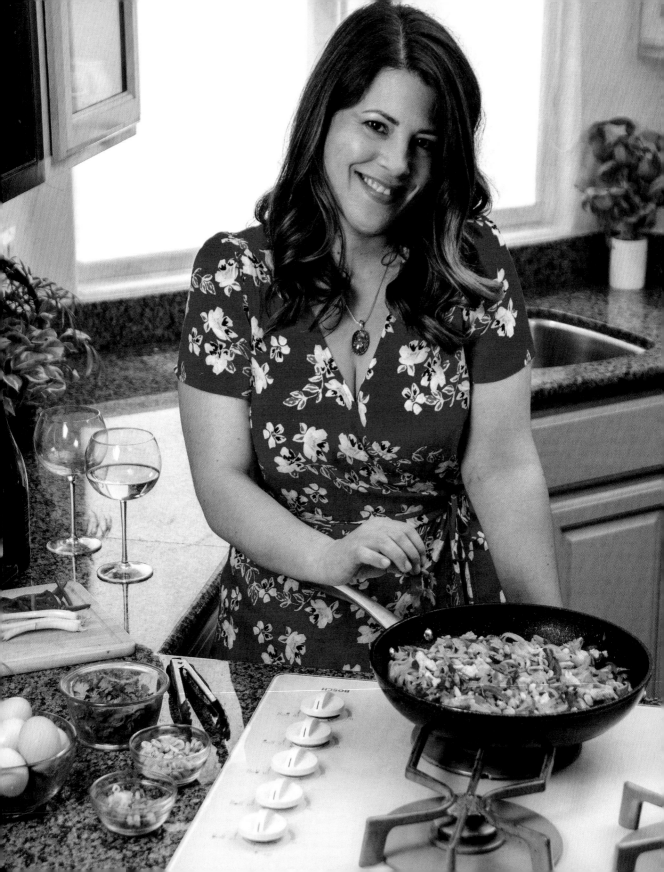

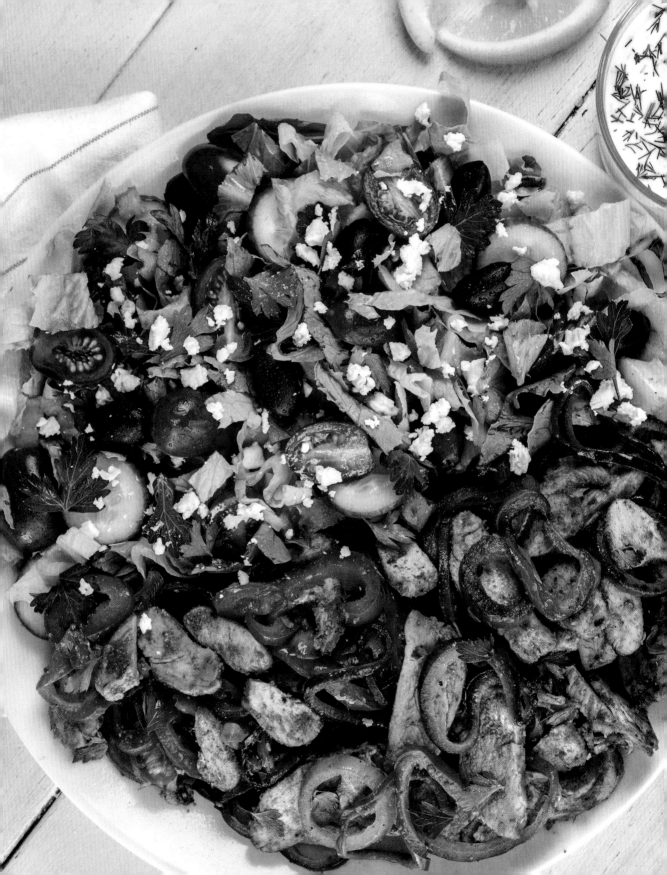

4. Meanwhile, make the yogurt sauce: In a small bowl, stir together the yogurt, lemon juice, dill, and celery salt. Thin with a little water to your preferred consistency and set aside.

5. Push the veggies to the sides of the skillet and add the chicken. Cook for 5 minutes on each side, or until cooked through and no longer pink in the center.

Remove the chicken from the pan and cut it into thin slices. Return the chicken to the skillet, along with any juices from the cutting board, and toss to combine. Remove from the heat.

6. Serve the chicken and veggies over the mixed greens, topped with the yogurt sauce.

Stovetop Chicken Parmesan

Here's another shortcut recipe! I love chicken Parmesan, but I don't always love all the work it takes to make it. This recipe simplifies the process: You cut the chicken into thinner pieces so you don't have to pound it flat or transfer it from the pan to the oven. I know these seem like easy enough steps, but when you're trying to get dinner on the table, every minute counts!

◯ **SERVING SIZE:** 1 chicken cutlet and ½ cup spinach   **PREP TIME:** 5 minutes   **COOK TIME:** 25 minutes
PER SERVING: *calories 254; fat 9 g; saturated fat 3.5 g; fiber 2 g; protein 22 g; carbohydrates 20 g; sugar 5 g*

1 (4-ounce) boneless, skinless chicken breast
⅓ cup panko bread crumbs (regular or gluten free)
3 tablespoons freshly grated Parmesan cheese
Pinch of kosher salt
Pinch of freshly ground black pepper
1 large egg
Olive oil spray
⅓ cup Marinara Sauce (page 103) or your favorite all-natural store-bought sauce
¼ cup shredded mozzarella cheese
1 cup baby spinach

1. Place the chicken breast on a cutting board and, using a small sharp knife, slice horizontally into the fatter side of the breast and cut all the way through to make 2 thin cutlets. (Place your hand on the top of the chicken breast as you cut through to steady it.)

2. In a shallow bowl or pie pan, combine the panko, Parmesan, salt, and pepper. In another bowl or pie pan, whisk the egg.

3. Spray a large skillet with olive oil and heat it over medium heat.

4. Dunk a chicken cutlet in the egg, dredge it in the panko, then set it on a plate. Repeat to coat the second cutlet.

5. Place the chicken in the preheated pan and cook on one side for 10 minutes, or until lightly browned on the bottom. Turn the chicken over. Spoon the marinara sauce evenly over both pieces of chicken and sprinkly them evenly with the mozzarella. Cover and cook for 10 to 15 minutes, until the chicken is cooked through and the mozzarella is nicely melted.

6. Serve on a bed of baby spinach.

KID-FAVORITE MEALS
ADULTS WILL LOVE

'm one of those lucky parents whose kid loves food and cooking. Well, part of it is luck and part of it is upbringing. Since she was two, Sophia has been watching me cook, and she started helping shortly thereafter. Now, at eleven, she makes entire dinners!

The best tip I can give you to get your kids enthusiastic about cooking and food is to let them passively watch. Homework is the perfect activity for this if you have school-age kids. Set your kids up at the kitchen counter to do their homework as you make dinner. You'll be spending time together, and they will inadvertently learn more about food and cooking.

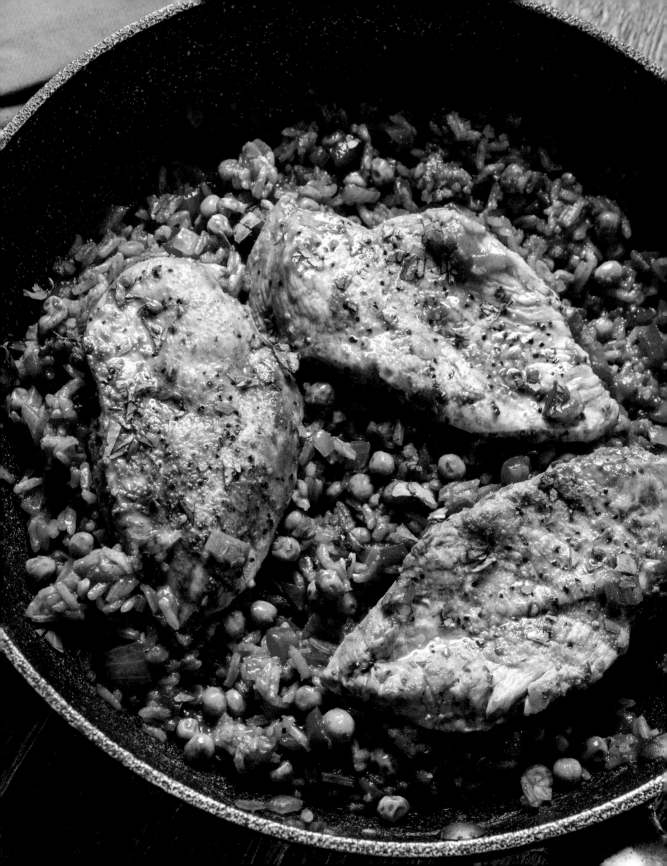

Arroz con Pollo

Arroz con pollo (chicken with rice) is a great family meal, and one that my daughter loves dearly.

Make this family-friendly meal for everyone, or make a big batch just for the kids. Then they can enjoy leftovers all week while you have more grown-up meals.

⭕ **SERVING SIZE:** 1 chicken cutlet and 1 cup rice   **COOK TIME:** 30 minutes   **PREP TIME:** 5 minutes
PER SERVING: *calories 311; fat 3 g; saturated fat 0.5 g; fiber 6 g; protein 15 g; carbohydrates 56 g; sugar 11 g*

2 (4-ounce) boneless, skinless chicken
   breasts
¼ teaspoon kosher salt
¼ teaspoon freshly ground black pepper
1 teaspoon ground cumin
1 teaspoon garlic powder
⅛ teaspoon cayenne pepper (this
   won't make it very spicy, but adjust to
   your taste)
1½ cups low-sodium chicken broth
1 (15-ounce) can tomato sauce
1 teaspoon olive oil
1 medium yellow onion, cut into
   medium dice
2 bell peppers, cut into medium dice
   (red is most easily "hidden" in this recipe)
2 garlic cloves, minced
1 cup long-grain white rice
1 cup frozen peas
¼ cup roughly chopped fresh cilantro

1. Place a chicken breast on a cutting board and, using a small sharp knife, slice horizontally into the fatter side of the breast and cut all the way through to make 2 thin cutlets. (Place your hand on the top of the chicken breast as you cut through to steady it.) Repeat with the second breast.

2. Coat the chicken with the salt, black pepper, cumin, garlic powder, and cayenne. This doesn't have to be precise. Just try to divide the spices evenly among the chicken cutlets.

3. In a medium bowl, mix the chicken broth and tomato sauce.

4. In a large skillet with a lid, heat the oil over medium-high heat. Add the chicken, onion, and bell peppers and cook for 10 minutes, turning the chicken halfway through. Mix in the garlic and the rice and cook for 1 minute.

5. Add the broth–tomato sauce mixture to the pan, stir to combine, and move the chicken to the surface of the mixture. Bring to a simmer, reduce the heat to medium-low, cover, and cook for 20 minutes, undisturbed, until the rice is cooked through.

6. Uncover and add the peas. Remove from the heat, cover, and let sit for 5 minutes. Serve hot, topped with the cilantro.

Huevos Rancheros Tacos

These may be the best tacos I've ever made! Not only are they delicious, but they're easy to whip up in a flash.

Now, I don't usually call for store-bought salsa . . . but it makes this dish especially easy. Just be sure to get organic to help avoid added chemicals and preservatives. At my store, it was only $0.50 more than nonorganic salsa.

◯ **SERVING SIZE:** 2 tacos   **COOK TIME:** 15 minutes   **PREP TIME:** 1 minute
PER SERVING: *calories 435; fat 21 g; saturated fat 6 g; fiber 10 g; protein 21 g; carbohydrates 43 g; sugar 2.5 g*

Olive oil spray
1 (16-ounce) jar organic mild salsa
¼ cup canned black beans, drained and rinsed
4 large eggs
4 (5-inch) corn tortillas
1 tablespoon crumbled Cotija cheese
½ avocado, sliced

1. Spray a large skillet with olive oil and set it over medium heat. Add the salsa and beans and cook for 10 minutes, stirring often to avoid burning. When the mixture is thick and lightly browned, transfer it to a bowl and wipe out the skillet.

2. Increase the heat to medium-high and spray the skillet with olive oil. Crack the eggs gently into the pan and fry them for 5 to 8 minutes, to your desired doneness, working in batches as needed to avoid overcrowding.

3. Meanwhile, heat the tortillas in the microwave according to the package directions.

4. To assemble the tacos, place a tortilla on a plate and top it with some beans and salsa, an egg, some Cotija, and some avocado slices.

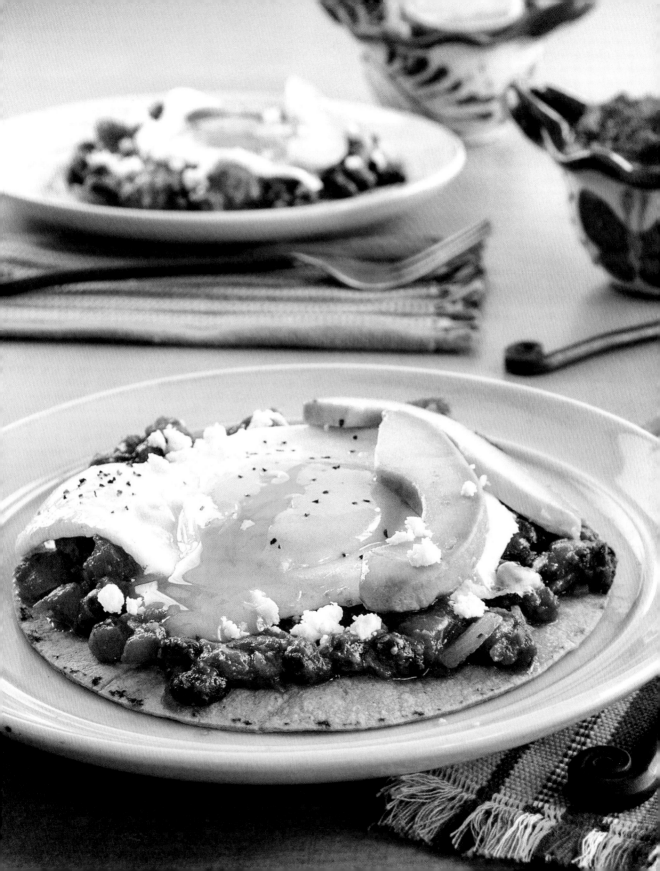

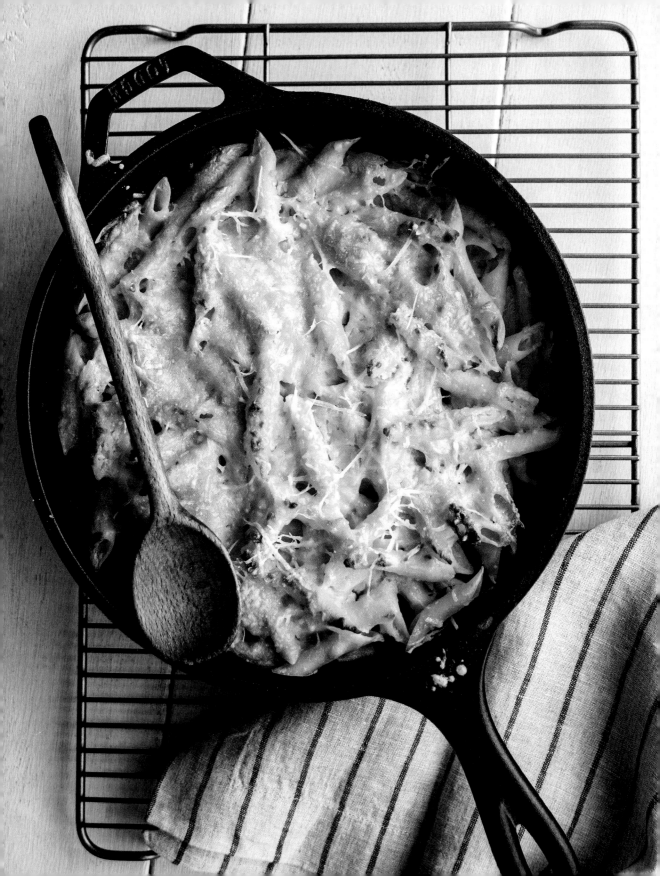

Butternut Squash Mac and Cheese

I have never been able to get my daughter to eat butternut squash . . . until now. When we tested this recipe, I made one batch of mac and cheese with butternut squash and one with sweet potato. I preferred the sweet potato (and you could easily make that here by swapping out the squash), but Sophia loved the butternut squash. She wanted the leftovers every day for dinner and still talks about the "orange mac and cheese."

If your kids are picky eaters, don't tell them there are vegetables in this recipe . . . just serve it with a smile.

⊙ **SERVING SIZE:** 1¼ cups   **COOK TIME:** 50 minutes   **PREP TIME:** 5 minutes
PER SERVING: *calories 210; fat 4 g; saturated fat 1.5 g; fiber 1 g; protein 9 g; carbohydrates 35 g; sugar 1 g*

---

1 (16-ounce) box penne pasta
2 cups 1-inch cubes butternut squash
2 cups unsweetened almond milk (or whatever unsweetened milk you have on hand)
½ cup low-sodium vegetable broth
½ cup shredded sharp cheddar cheese
Kosher salt and freshly ground black pepper

1. Preheat the oven to 400°F.

2. Bring a large pot of water to a boil. Add the penne and cook until al dente according to the package directions. Drain and set aside.

3. Meanwhile, in a large saucepan, combine the squash, almond milk, and broth. Cook over medium-high heat for 10 to 15 minutes, until the squash is soft.

4. Remove from the heat and use an immersion blender to blend the squash until smooth. (Alternatively, cool for 15 minutes, then use a traditional blender to blend the squash until smooth, but be sure to vent the top to avoid a hot explosion. Return to the saucepan.)

5. Mix the drained pasta and cheddar into the squash puree. Season with salt and pepper to taste.

6. Transfer the pasta to a 9 × 13-inch baking dish or large cast-iron skillet. Bake for 20 minutes, until hot and bubbling. Scoop into bowls and serve.

Pizza Quesadillas

These quesadillas are so easy and delicious, and I promise your kids will love them! The recipe makes one serving. I have one kid; perhaps you have two or more. Just do a bit of arithmetic and you can make as many as you like. . . . Hey, you could even make the kids do the math. Less work for you, math lesson for them!

What I love the most is that I can freeze all the ingredients, so you can buy them when they're on sale to stock up and save money. And yes, you can freeze shredded cheese.

◎ **SERVING SIZE:** 1 quesadilla   **COOK TIME:** 10 minutes   **PREP TIME:** 1 minute
PER SERVING: *calories 211; fat 6.5 g; saturated fat 2 g; fiber 1.5 g; protein 6 g; carbohydrates 33 g; sugar 2.5 g*

Olive oil spray
1 (10-inch) flour tortilla
¼ cup shredded mozzarella cheese
2 tablespoons tomato sauce

OPTIONAL TOPPINGS
Pepperoni (look for nitrate-free)
Cooked and crumbled sausage
Chopped bell peppers
Chopped mushrooms
Chopped red onion
Sliced olives
Chopped pineapple

1. Lightly spray a large skillet with olive oil and heat over medium heat.

2. Set the tortilla in the pan and top one side with the mozzarella, tomato sauce, and toppings of your choice. Fold the tortilla over. Cook for 5 minutes on each side, until the cheese is melted and the tortilla is golden brown.

3. Slice (I use scissors to make it easier) into 4 pieces and serve with your favorite toppings.

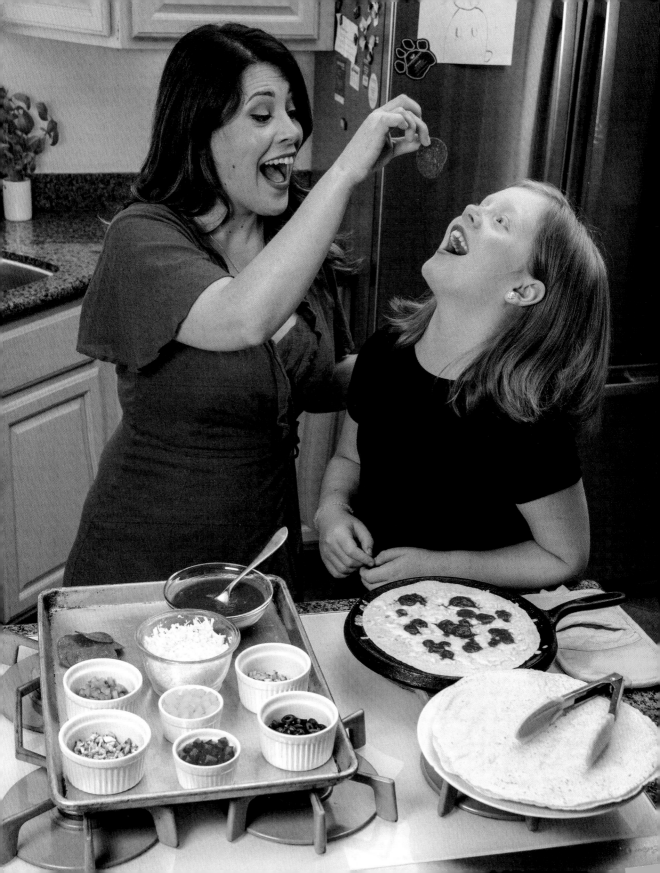

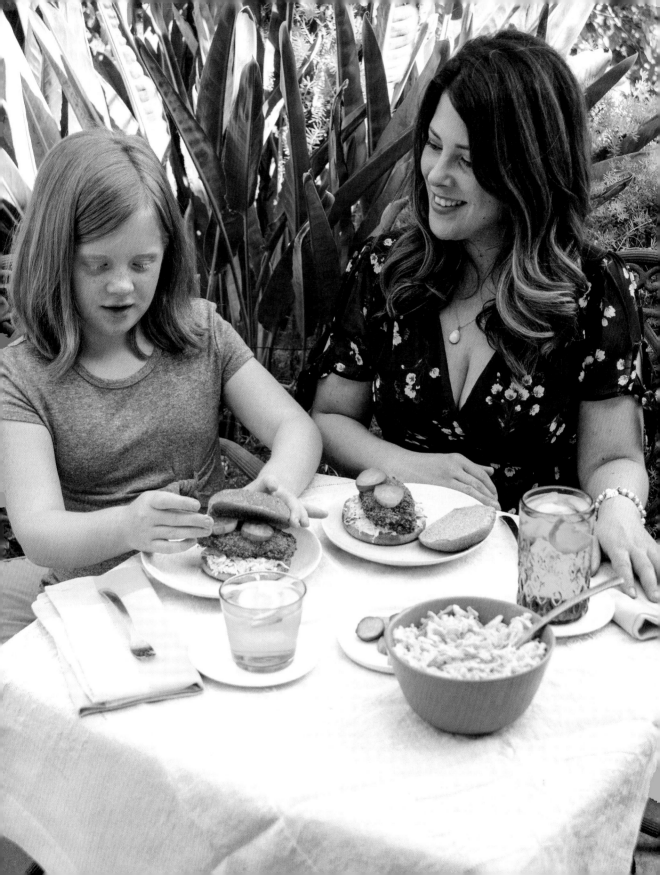

Cooking with Kids

Excuse me while I get up on my soapbox for a moment. . . . I strongly believe that we should be teaching our kids how to cook and how to eat healthy, starting at a very young age!

Most schools don't teach cooking or healthy eating, which leaves it to parents to lead the charge on all kitchen- and food-related lessons. And though that may seem burdensome, I believe if done right it can actually be a great bonding activity, and you may even find a pastime that you and your kids will enjoy doing together through their adult years!

I started teaching my daughter how to cook at age two, and now at eleven she can cook entire meals. She fixes herself breakfast on the weekends, allowing me some much-needed extra sleep. If you have teenagers and have not yet taught them any kitchen skills, don't fret. . . . I didn't learn how to cook until I was in my thirties, and look at me now. You can start teaching them right now, and they will pick it up fast!

Here are some lessons to try with your kids, whatever their ages.

Ages 1 to 3

- Helping you *measure* ingredients, or *adding* premeasured ingredients for younger cooks
- Cracking eggs (do it into a clean, empty bowl; it makes fishing for shells easier)
- Mixing dry ingredients together
- Anything with the rolling pin
- Cutting out cookies and decorating them

Ages 4 to 6

- Using the toaster
- Assembly jobs (such as prepping Pizza Quesadillas, page 72)
- Measuring ingredients for you
- Using a butter knife to spread

Ages 7 to 10

- Stovetop cooking, with adult supervision
- Making rice, pasta, and similar dishes
- Reading and following recipe directions
- Handling meat (start with cooked and work your way to raw)

Ages 11 to 14

- Using electric mixers
- Introducing sharp objects with supervision, such as pizza cutters and kitchen scissors
- Cleaning and washing produce
- Washing up after cooking!

Ages 15 to 18

- Oven use, supervised at first
- Proper knife handling, supervised, of course
- Blender and food processor use
- Grilling safety and proper use (for the older kids—keep a close eye if there's an open flame!)

Before I leave you to your cooking lessons, I have one more thing for you to think about. Even if your kids don't want to learn, you can lead by example. I don't send my daughter to her room to do her homework; instead she does it at the kitchen counter. Or if she wants to play computer games after school, I set her up at the kitchen counter. This way she learns by passively watching. I've seen the benefits of her being in the same room with me while I work grow over the years, from her general knowledge of food and nutrition to how to make some meals. Try this approach for your more reluctant kitchen students.

Cheeseburger Mac and Cheese

Friends . . . this may sound strange, but trust me, it's amazing! Plus, it's one of my daughter's favorite dinners ever.

I like to make a big batch of this for her lunches during summer, or for weeknight dinners when I know I'll be making more grown-up meals for myself. It holds well in the fridge, and you can divide it into individual portions and freeze them for homemade freezer meals.

SERVING SIZE: 1½ cups **COOK TIME:** 30 minutes **PREP TIME:** 5 minutes
PER SERVING: *calories 470; fat 8 g; saturated fat 2 g; fiber 5.5 g; protein 24 g; carbohydrates 75 g; sugar 12 g*

---

1 (16-ounce) box penne pasta or elbow macaroni
1 medium red onion, diced
1 pound lean ground turkey or bison
1 tablespoon all-purpose flour
2 cups unsweetened almond milk (or whatever unsweetened milk you have on hand)
1 to 2 teaspoons yellow mustard, to taste
½ cup shredded sharp cheddar cheese
2 tablespoons sliced dill pickles
20 cherry tomatoes, halved

1. Preheat the oven to 400°F.

2. Bring a large pot of water to a boil. Add the pasta and cook until al dente according to the package directions. Drain and set aside.

3. Meanwhile, in a large skillet, combine the onion and turkey over medium heat, breaking the turkey into large chunks. Cook for about 5 minutes, or until the turkey is browned and the onion is soft. Transfer the mixture to a plate, leaving 1 tablespoon of the fat in the pan.

4. Reduce the heat to low and add the flour. Mix in a figure-eight to make a roux. After about 2 minutes, when the roux is browned and no longer smells of flour, add the milk and whisk well to incorporate. Cook for 10 minutes, whisking often, until thickened, then mix in the mustard. Mix in the drained pasta, the cooked turkey, most of the cheddar, and the pickles.

5. Transfer the pasta mixture to a 9 × 13-inch baking dish. Sprinkle the remaining cheddar and the tomatoes on top and bake for 15 minutes, or until the cheese is melted and the sauce is bubbling. Serve hot.

ONE POT, PAN, DISH, OR SHEET

'm a lazy cook, and I'm not afraid to admit it. I hate cleaning up almost as much as I hate a dirty kitchen. So I love one-pan dishes that are easy to prepare and clean up.

All the recipes in this book are easy, but these recipes take it a step further and also make cleanup a breeze.

Apple Sage Chicken

I love easy one-pan meals. Mostly because I don't like to do a lot of dishes . . . but also because of the ease of tossing everything into one pan and walking away.

This recipe is great with all boneless cuts of chicken or boneless pork chops (bone-in will take more time to cook and slightly change the flavor), so try it with whatever boneless protein you have available. Hey, it's all about ease in this recipe!

◎ **SERVING SIZE:** 1 chicken breast and half the apples **PREP TIME:** 2 minutes **COOK TIME:** 25 minutes
PER SERVING: *calories 467; fat 7 g; saturated fat 0.5 g; fiber 4 g; protein 78 g; carbohydrates 23 g; sugar 17 g*

---

1 teaspoon olive oil
2 (4-ounce) boneless, skinless
 chicken breasts
Pinch of kosher salt
Pinch of freshly ground black pepper
½ teaspoon pumpkin pie spice
2 green apples, cored and cut into
 medium slices
1 fresh sage sprig

1. In a large skillet, heat the oil over medium-low heat.

2. Lightly sprinkle the chicken on both sides with the salt, pepper, and pumpkin pie spice. Place the chicken in the center of the hot pan and surround it with the apples. Top with the sage and cook for 12 minutes, or until browned on the bottom.

3. Flip the chicken, stir the apples, cover, and cook for 10 to 12 minutes, until the chicken is cooked through and no longer pink in the center and the apples are soft.

4. Discard the sage and top the chicken with the apples to serve.

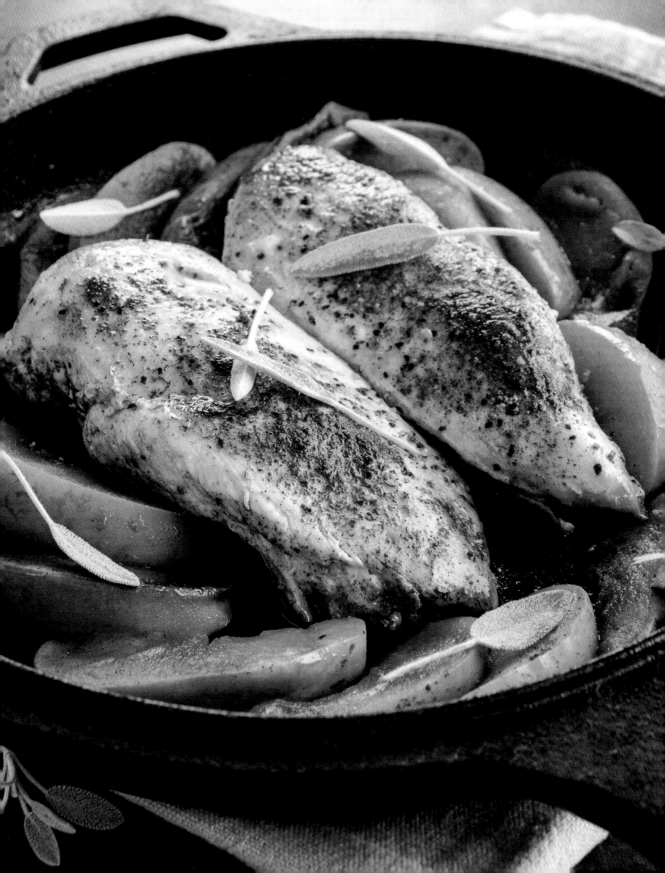

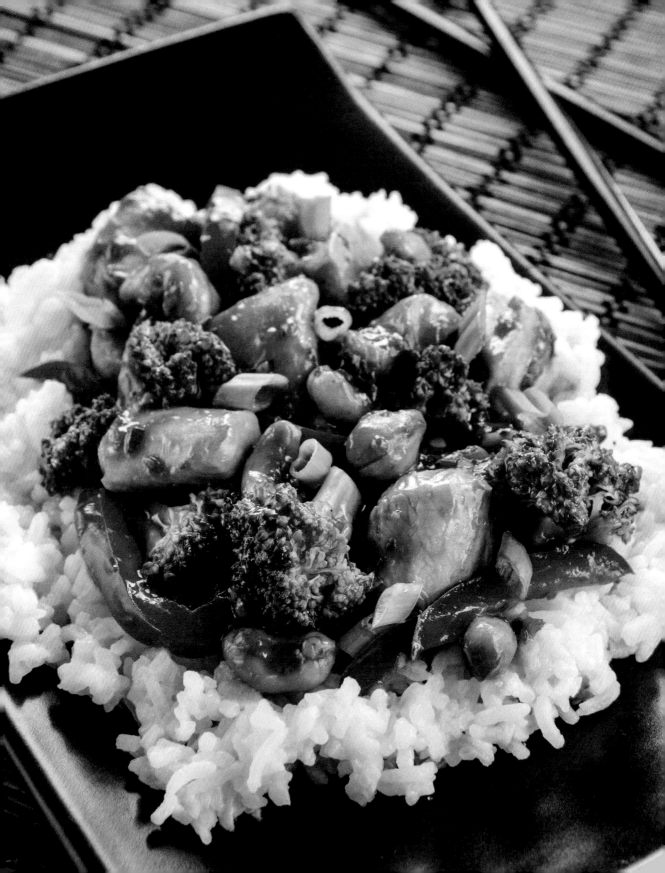

Cashew Chicken

🥫 MAKES 4 SERVINGS

Here's a 15-minute dinner to the rescue. Easy to make, easy to clean up, and completely delicious.

I couldn't find unsalted cashews the last time I went to the store, so I rinsed some salted cashews and it turned out great. Be sure to do the same if you are using salted cashews, as this is already a pretty salty dish with the soy sauce and chili garlic sauce.

○ **SERVING SIZE:** about 1 cup **PREP TIME:** 5 minutes **COOK TIME:** 15 minutes
PER SERVING: *calories 302; fat 14.5 g; saturated fat 3 g; fiber 2.5 g; protein 25 g; carbohydrates 20 g; sugar 7.5 g*

2 tablespoons soy sauce (or tamari, for a gluten-free dish)
1 tablespoon honey
1½ teaspoons rice vinegar
1 tablespoon chili garlic sauce
1 teaspoon ground ginger
2 tablespoons cornstarch
1 teaspoon toasted sesame oil or olive oil
2 (4-ounce) boneless, skinless chicken breasts, cut into 1-inch cubes
2 cups broccoli florets
1 red bell pepper, diced
2 garlic cloves, minced
½ cup unsalted cashews
2 green onions, thinly sliced

1. In a medium bowl, combine the soy sauce, honey, vinegar, chili garlic sauce, ginger, and cornstarch. Set the sauce aside.

2. In a large skillet, heat the sesame oil over medium heat. Add the chicken and cook for 5 minutes, stirring occasionally to brown all sides. Transfer to a plate (it's okay if the chicken isn't fully cooked).

3. Add the broccoli, bell pepper, and garlic to the pan. Cover and cook, undisturbed, for 5 minutes.

4. Uncover the pan and add the sauce, cashews, and chicken (along with any juices on the plate). Stir to combine. Cook for 3 to 5 minutes, until the chicken is cooked through and the sauce has thickened.

5. Top with the green onions and serve hot.

One Pot, Pan, Dish, or Sheet

Greek Chicken and Rice

Before you get started on this recipe, find your best skillet with a lid. You want one with a good seal so that the rice can cook properly.

Now let me rave about this dish. It's just as good hot out of the pan as it is served cold over some mixed greens the next day. So, if you're looking to save some time or money on tomorrow's lunch, double this recipe and take the leftovers with you for lunch this week. I like to chop the leftover chicken before putting it in a storage container, making my salad prep the next day a little easier. Oh, and the Greek dressing from Simple Greek Salad (page 21) is amazing with this!

SERVING SIZE: 1 chicken cutlet and ½ cup rice   **COOK TIME:** 30 minutes   **PREP TIME:** 5 minutes
PER SERVING: *calories 406; fat 9.5 g; saturated fat 1 g; fiber 3 g; protein 31 g; carbohydrates 47 g; sugar 4.5 g*

1½ teaspoons olive oil
½ medium red onion, diced
1 red bell pepper, diced
Pinch of kosher salt
Pinch of freshly ground black pepper
1 (4-ounce) boneless, skinless
  chicken breast
3 garlic cloves, minced
½ cup long-grain white rice
8 Kalamata olives, pitted and quartered
1 teaspoon minced fresh dill
1 cup baby spinach
Juice of 1 lemon
½ teaspoon ground cumin
1 cup low-sodium chicken broth

1. In a large skillet, heat the oil over medium heat. Add the onion, bell pepper, salt, and black pepper and sauté for 5 minutes, stirring often to avoid burning.

2. Meanwhile, place the chicken breast on a cutting board and, using a small sharp knife, slice horizontally into the fatter side of the breast and cut all the way through to make 2 thin cutlets. (Place your hand on the top of the chicken breast as you cut through to steady it.)

3. Add the garlic and rice to the vegetables in the skillet and stir to combine. Mix in the olives, dill, spinach, lemon juice, cumin, and broth. Place the chicken on top of the mixture, cover the pan tightly, reduce the heat to medium-low, and cook, undisturbed, for 25 minutes, until the rice and chicken are fully cooked.

4. Serve hot, and save any leftovers for a salad tomorrow . . . yum!

Fried Rice

For fried rice, you want to use cold cooked rice. So, make your life easy and cook the rice the night before, or purchase precooked rice (look in the freezer section). Dinner will be ready in just 10 minutes.

To make this a vegan dish, use ¼ cup crumbled firm or extra-firm tofu in place of the eggs.

○ **SERVING SIZE:** ½ cup   **PREP TIME:** 5 minutes   **COOK TIME:** 12 minutes
PER SERVING: *calories 202; fat 3 g; saturated fat 1 g; fiber 2.5 g; protein 7 g; carbohydrates 37 g; sugar 3 g*

1 teaspoon toasted sesame oil
1 medium onion, cut into medium chunks
2 garlic cloves, minced
2 cups cooked rice
2 large eggs
1½ cups frozen peas and carrots, thawed
2 tablespoons soy sauce (or tamari, for a gluten-free meal)
2 green onions, thickly sliced

1. In a large skillet or wok, heat the sesame oil over medium-high heat. Add the onion and cook for 5 minutes, stirring often. Add the garlic and cook for 1 minute.

2. Add the rice and cook, undisturbed, for 5 minutes, then push the mixture to the sides of the skillet. Crack the eggs into the pan and quickly whisk them with a wooden spoon. Once the eggs are set, mix in the peas and carrots, soy sauce, rice, and green onions. Serve hot.

Shakshuka

This is one of my favorite dinners to make on a weeknight. It's easy and fast and, because it's just Sophia and me, we have leftovers for breakfast . . . and let me tell you, this dish makes for a great breakfast!

I like to serve it with pitas, cut into quarters. It's a nice sauce-mopping device that goes really well with this yummy dish.

SERVING SIZE: 1 egg, ¼ cup tomato sauce, and 2 tablespoons yogurt sauce
PREP TIME: 5 minutes   **COOK TIME:** 25 minutes
PER SERVING: *calories 136; fat 7 g; saturated fat 2 g; fiber 1.5 g; protein 12 g; carbohydrates 8 g; sugar 5.5 g*

YOGURT SAUCE
½ cup 0% Greek yogurt
¼ teaspoon garlic salt
¼ teaspoon chopped fresh dill

SHAKSHUKA
1 teaspoon olive oil
1 medium onion, sliced
1 red bell pepper, thinly sliced
Pinch of kosher salt
Pinch of freshly ground black pepper
4 garlic cloves, minced
1 teaspoon ground cumin
1 teaspoon paprika
⅛ teaspoon cayenne pepper
1 (28-ounce) can diced tomatoes
4 large eggs
2 tablespoons crumbled feta cheese
⅓ cup roughly chopped fresh flat-leaf parsley

1. Make the yogurt sauce: In a medium bowl, whisk together the yogurt, garlic salt, dill, and 1 tablespoon water. Set aside.

2. Make the shakshuka: In a large skillet, heat the oil over medium heat. Add the onion, bell pepper, salt, and black pepper. Cover and cook for 5 minutes, stirring once or twice to avoid burning, until soft. Uncover, stir, add the garlic, and cook for 2 minutes.

3. Stir in the cumin, paprika, and cayenne. Add the tomatoes, increase the heat to medium-high, cover, and cook for 15 minutes, until bubbling.

4. Stir the mixture, then make four wells in it and crack an egg into each well. Cover and cook for 3 minutes for runny yolks, 4 to 5 minutes for set yolks. Uncover and remove from the heat, sprinkle the feta and parsley over the top, and serve with the yogurt sauce.

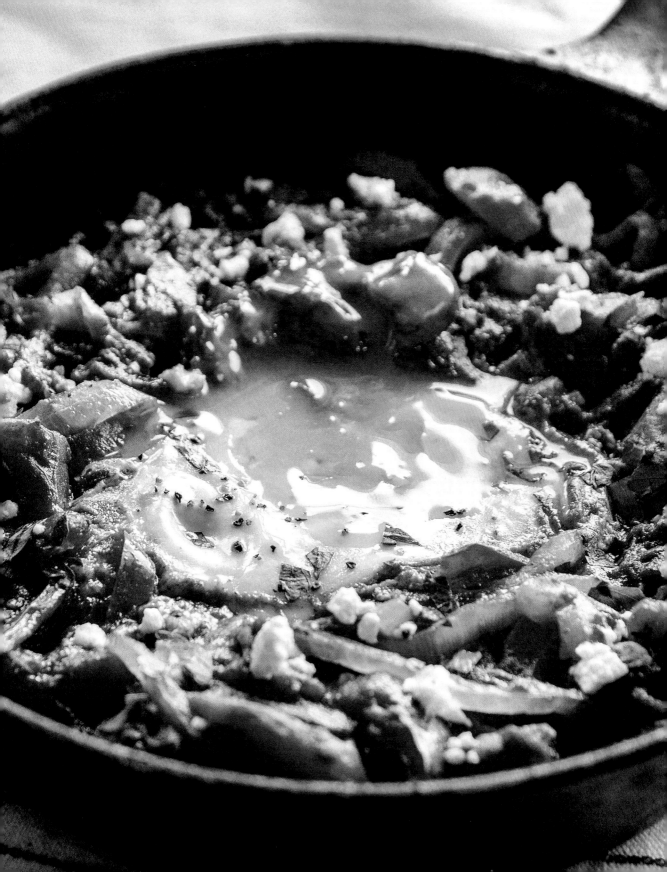

ONCE-A-WEEK COOKING

had a chapter similar to this in my cookbook *Lose Weight with Your Instant Pot*. I said it there and I'll say it here . . . one day I'll write an entire cookbook on once-a-week cooking. This is how I cook when I'm not recipe testing. I make a big Sunday dinner (with marinara sauce or roasted chicken, for example) and then repurpose the leftovers from the large prep recipes into quick meals for the rest of the week.

Shredded Citrus Chicken

🥫 MAKES 8 SERVINGS

Here it is, the token whole chicken recipe. Every cookbook I've written has included a whole chicken recipe. It's my favorite thing to make, ever!

In this version I use salt rather than oil to make the skin crispy. If you're trying to lower your salt intake, simply replace it with olive oil spray.

I've included two different options for prepping the chicken here. Both ways are delicious! You might try the easy way the first time you make the chicken and the more advanced method when you've gained a bit of kitchen confidence. The advanced method will yield a more flavorful chicken, and will look more impressive as well.

I like to use this shredded chicken in Curried Chicken Salad (page 94).

SERVING SIZE: 4 ounces   **PREP TIME:** 5 minutes (easy) or 15 minutes (advanced)   **COOK TIME:** 2 hours
PER SERVING: *calories 103; fat 5 g; saturated fat 1.5 g; fiber 0.5 g; protein 10 g; carbohydrates 3 g; sugar 2 g*

---

1 (5-pound) whole chicken
5 garlic cloves
3 fresh thyme sprigs
3 oranges, 3 lemons, or a combo of both
   (I like 2 oranges and 1 lemon)
1½ teaspoons kosher salt

1. Preheat the oven to 350°F.

2. Place the chicken in a roasting pan. Check the cavity and neck for extra pieces. The heart and giblets can be used to make chicken stock and the liver can be cooked for a chef's treat or for your pets! In any event, remove them from the bird.

3. **EASY PREP METHOD:** Place the garlic cloves and thyme inside the chicken cavity. Cut each piece of citrus into 8 round slices and add to the pan, shoving a few inside the

chicken. Sprinkle the chicken evenly with the salt.

ADVANCED PREP METHOD: Use a rasp-style grater to zest the citrus into a small bowl. Use the same grater to grate 1 clove of the garlic and add it to the bowl with the zest. Mince the leaves from 1 sprig of thyme and add them to the bowl. Mix together.

Slide your fingers (or hands, if you have small hands like me) under the skin on the chicken breasts to separate the skin from the meat. Reach farther in to do the same on the thighs and legs to the best of your ability. Spread the zest-garlic mixture evenly under the skin.

Add the remaining garlic and thyme to the chicken cavity. Cut each piece of citrus into 8 wedges and pack them into the cavity until it is packed. Drop the remaining citrus wedges into the pan. Sprinkle the chicken evenly with the salt. Truss the legs together with kitchen twine and fold the wings back so they don't burn.

4. Set the chicken in a shallow roasting pan. Roast the chicken for about 2 hours, until the internal temperature is 165°F in the thickest part of the breast, the juices run clear, and the skin is golden brown, basting the outside and inside two or three times with the drippings. Let rest for 30 minutes before shredding.

5. Store leftovers in the fridge for up to 4 days, or in the freezer for 1 to 2 months. I like to divide the leftovers into 1-cup portions freezer bags or storage containers for easy measuring later.

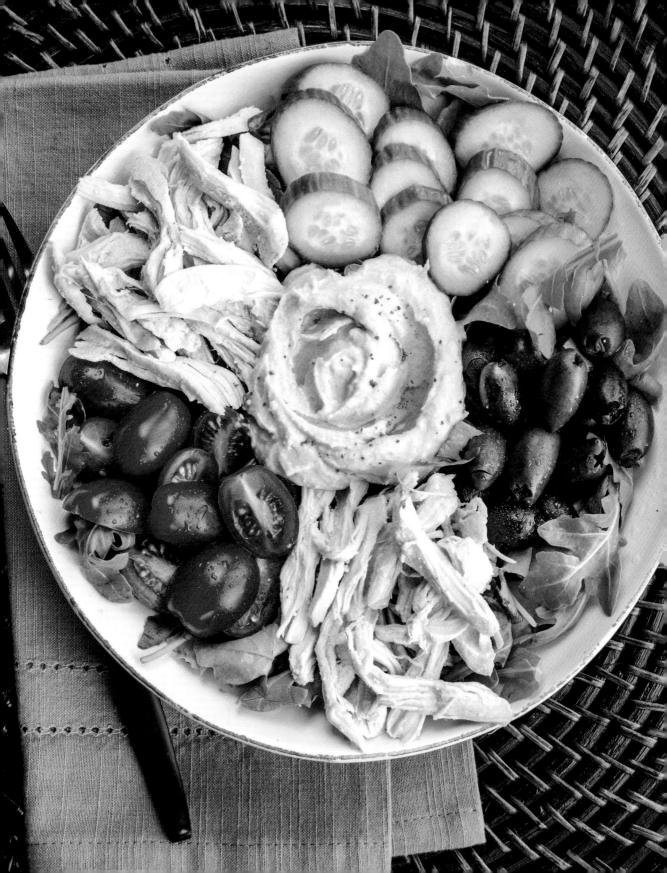

Hummus Bowl

Here's a healthy way to indulge in your favorite snack at mealtime. Use leftover Shredded Citrus Chicken (page 90) in this quick and easy dinner.

You could easily make this a vegan meal by leaving out the chicken. I've often done it myself! Whether you're a vegan or not, it's a great way to save money.

◎ **SERVING SIZE:** ⅓ cup hummus, 1 cup greens, and toppings   **PREP TIME:** 5 minutes   **COOK TIME:** 0 minutes
PER SERVING: *calories 415; fat 8.5 g; saturated fat 1.5 g; fiber 19 g; protein 24 g; carbohydrates 65 g; sugar 23 g*

---

1 (15-ounce) can chickpeas (garbanzo beans), undrained

1 tablespoon olive oil

1 teaspoon tahini

1 teaspoon fresh lemon juice

1 garlic clove

¼ teaspoon kosher salt

¼ teaspoon freshly ground black pepper

4 cups mixed greens (about a 5-ounce package)

1 cup Shredded Citrus Chicken (page 90)

1 (10-ounce) container grape tomatoes

1 English cucumber, cut into medium slices

10 Kalamata olives, pitted and sliced into thin rings

1. Drain the liquid from the can of chickpeas into a small bowl and set aside. In a blender, combine the chickpeas, oil, tahini, lemon juice, garlic, salt, pepper, and half the canned chickpea liquid and blend until smooth, adding more of the chickpea liquid as desired to reach your preferred hummus consistency.

2. To serve, divide the greens among four plates and top evenly with the hummus, chicken, tomatoes, cucumber, and olives. Serve at room temperature or chilled out of the fridge—it's good both ways.

Curried Chicken Salad

Chicken salad is such a great way to repurpose leftover chicken. Make this with Shredded Citrus Chicken (page 90). The curry powder changes the flavor profile and adds complexity.

I like to serve this several different ways, depending on what I have available in the house. My favorite way to enjoy it is as a wrap in a spinach tortilla with some mixed greens and tomatoes, but usually I simply add it to a plate of mixed greens. It's also great on toast or wrapped in butter lettuce or romaine leaves in place of bready carbs.

SERVING SIZE: 1½ cups **PREP TIME:** 5 minutes **COOK TIME:** 0 minutes
PER SERVING: *calories 192; fat 6 g; saturated fat 1 g; fiber 2.5 g; protein 22 g; carbohydrates 13 g; sugar 9 g*

---

1 cup Shredded Citrus Chicken (page 90)
1 celery stalk, minced
½ apple, cored and cut into ¼-inch chunks
1 tablespoon minced fresh chives
1 tablespoon raisins
1 tablespoon slivered almonds
½ teaspoon curry powder
¼ cup 0% Greek yogurt
Kosher salt and freshly ground black pepper

1. In a medium bowl, combine the chicken, celery, apple, chives, raisins, almonds, curry powder, and yogurt. Mix in salt and pepper to taste.

2. Serve over greens, in a wrap, or any way you like!

Carne Asada

I like to make this in bulk, so I buy enough ingredients for three batches of the recipe. I divide the steak into three 1-gallon freezer bags, then I divide the marinade into the bags with the steak and put one bag in the fridge to marinate for dinner that night and two bags into the freezer for another night. Why not make things easier for myself? I'm going to have the blender out anyway, and this means I have to clean it only once. When I pull out the frozen steak on another night, I feel a wave of gratitude toward past Audrey.

Try out Gringa Tacos (page 99)—it's a delicious way to use up your Carne Asada.

◯ **SERVING SIZE:** 2 ounces   **PREP TIME:** 5 minutes   **COOK TIME:** 20 minutes
PER SERVING: *calories 137; fat 6.5 g; saturated fat 2.5 g; fiber 0.5 g; protein 15 g; carbohydrates 3 g; sugar 2 g*

1 tablespoon olive oil
Juice of 2 limes
Juice of 2 oranges
4 garlic cloves
1 cup fresh cilantro sprigs
1 jalapeño
2 tablespoons distilled white vinegar
Pinch of kosher salt
Pinch of freshly ground black pepper
2 pounds skirt steak

1. In a blender, combine the oil, lime juice, orange juice, garlic, cilantro, jalapeño, vinegar, salt, and pepper and blend until smooth. Transfer the marinade to a resealable gallon bag. Add the steak, seal the bag, and marinate in the fridge for at least 2 hours and up to 24 hours.

2. Preheat a grill to high heat.

3. Remove the steak from the marinade (discard the marinade). Grill the steak for 7 to 10 minutes on each side, until it reaches your desired doneness. Let the steak rest for 10 minutes, then slice and serve.

4. Store leftovers in the fridge for up to 4 days, or in the freezer for 1 to 2 months. I like to divide the leftovers into 1-cup portions freezer bags or storage containers for easy measuring later.

Individual Nachos

Nachos always sound like such a huge splurge, so when my friend Heidi and her kids, Ethan and Andy, came over one night, I knew these would be a huge hit! Everyone loved them, and Heidi and I both piled our nachos high with jalapeños and avocado . . . talk about a yummy dinner!

These mess-free nachos ensure that everyone gets their fair share of toppings. Plus, with the optional toppings, you can each spice yours up however you like. To make this easy dinner vegetarian, omit the Carne Asada and double the beans.

SERVING SIZE: 2 nachos   **PREP TIME:** 4 minutes   **COOK TIME:** 5 minutes
PER SERVING: *calories 354; fat 16 g; saturated fat 7 g; fiber 5.5 g; protein 15 g; carbohydrates 37 g; sugar 1.5 g*

---

8 tostada shells
½ cup canned black beans, drained
    and rinsed
½ cup chopped Carne Asada (page 95)
½ cup shredded sharp cheddar cheese
½ cup finely diced red bell pepper
½ cup canned sliced black olives

OPTIONAL TOPPINGS
Pickled jalapeños
¼ cup diced red onion
0% Greek yogurt (in place of sour
    cream, yum!)
Diced avocado
Salsa
A squeeze of fresh lime juice

1. Preheat the oven to 350°F.

2. On one or two sheet pans, spread out the tostada shells so they're not overlapping. Top with the beans, carne asada, and cheddar, dividing them evenly. Bake for 5 minutes, or until the cheese is melted.

3. Top the nachos with the bell pepper, olives, and any other toppings you desire. (I like to add pickled jalapeños, red onion, and Greek yogurt.)

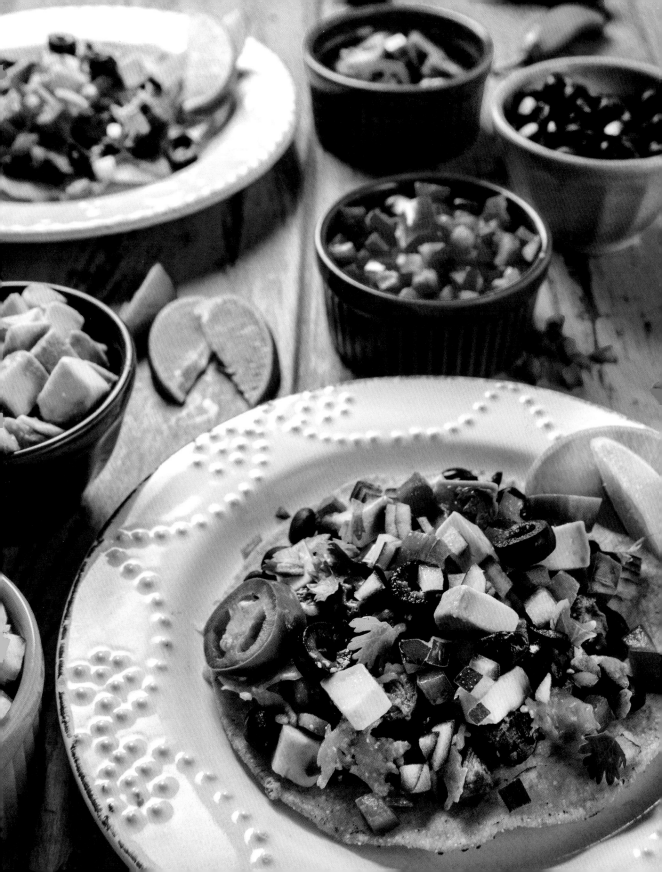

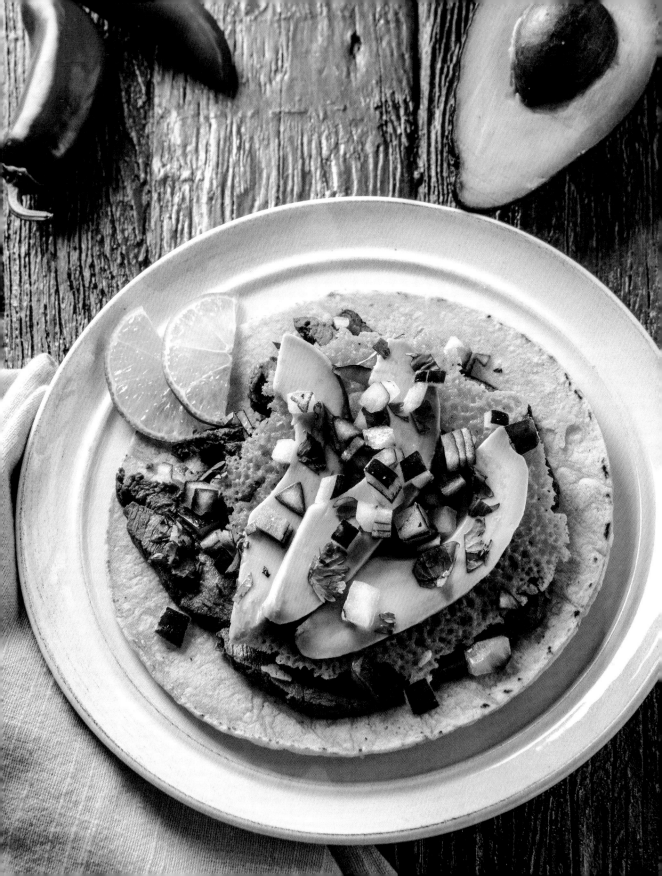

Gringa Tacos

There's a taco place Sophia and I love to frequent in downtown Boise. They make lots of different tacos, but we both prefer their Gringa Tacos. Now, the restaurant that makes them (Calle 75 Street Tacos) tops them with a fantastic habanero salsa. It's *H.O.T.* and I love it . . . but it's not for everyone, so just use your favorite hot sauce.

This recipe is a great way to use Carne Asada (page 95).

It's the melted cheese that makes these special, so don't just toss on some cold shredded cheese. It's so worth the tiny bit of extra cooking.

◯ **SERVING SIZE:** 2 tacos   **PREP TIME:** 3 minutes   **COOK TIME:** 5 minutes
PER SERVING: *calories 353; fat 17 g; saturated fat 9 g; fiber 3.5 g; protein 23 g; carbohydrates 25 g; sugar 2 g*

½ cup shredded sharp cheddar cheese
½ cup chopped Carne Asada (page 95)
4 corn tortillas
¼ cup chopped fresh cilantro
¼ cup minced red onion

OPTIONAL TOPPINGS
Hot sauce
Pickled or fresh jalapeño slices
Sliced avocado
0% Greek yogurt (instead of sour cream)

1. Heat a large skillet, preferably nonstick, over medium-high heat. Make 4 mounds of cheddar (2 tablespoons each) in the skillet, spaced so they don't merge as they melt. Cook for 5 minutes, until about 50 percent crispy.

2. Meanwhile, heat the tortillas according to the package directions and reheat the carne asada in the microwave for 1 minute or in a small skillet, covered, over medium-low heat for 3 minutes.

3. As soon as the cheese is 50 percent crispy, it's time to assemble . . . you don't want burnt cheese. To assemble, divide the meat among the tortillas, then scoop the cheddar crisps off the skillet and place them crispy side up over the meat. Top with the cilantro and red onion and serve with your favorite toppings.

Rigatoni with Vodka Sauce

I was up late one night thinking about this book and how I was going to make this classic pasta recipe healthy by getting rid of the heavy cream. Then the answer came to me . . . and it was the answer to almost every Lose Weight by Eating question (well, not really . . . but go with me here): *Greek yogurt!*

At first I was concerned that the yogurt would separate, but I had the idea to add it to the top of the pasta, where it would slowly heat up, instead of letting it curdle in the hot sauce, which would ruin the creamy consistency. Right out of the gate, this recipe was complete perfection!

This recipe works with leftover Marinara Sauce (page 103).

SERVING SIZE: 1 cup   **PREP TIME:** 1 minute   **COOK TIME:** 15 minutes
PER SERVING: *calories 354; fat 6.5 g; saturated fat 3 g; fiber 4.5 g; protein 13 g; carbohydrates 57 g; sugar 10.5 g*

---

1 (16-ounce) box rigatoni pasta
2 cups Marinara Sauce (page 103)
½ teaspoon red pepper flakes
2 tablespoons vodka
¼ cup 0% Greek yogurt
¼ cup freshly grated Parmesan cheese
¼ cup fresh basil leaves

1. Bring a large pot of water to a boil. Add the rigatoni and cook until al dente according to the package directions. Drain and set aside.

2. Meanwhile, in a large skillet, bring the marinara to a simmer over medium-high heat. Cook for 5 minutes, then stir in the red pepper flakes and vodka and remove from the heat.

3. Add the drained pasta to the sauce. Top with the yogurt and half the Parmesan, then mix together quickly to incorporate the yogurt and cheese.

4. Serve topped with the remaining Parmesan and the basil.

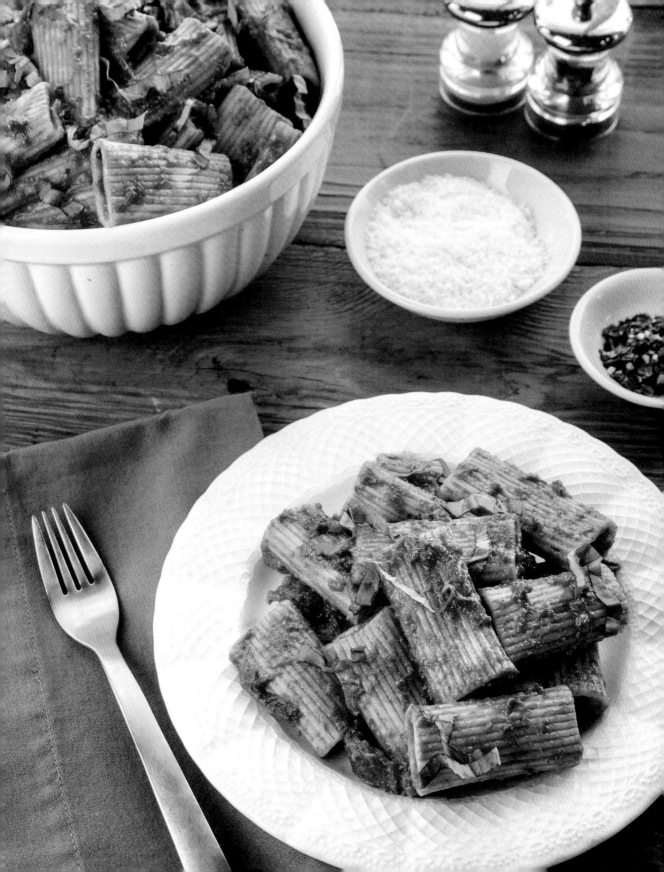

Fast French Bread Pizzas

MAKES 6 SERVINGS

This recipe is based on the Vegetarian French Bread Pizza in *Lose Weight by Eating: Detox Week*. In that book I hollow out the bread, but I thought this way would yield more servings and, therefore, save you money.

This fast dinner uses Marinara Sauce (page 103).

SERVING SIZE: ½ French bread pizza   **PREP TIME:** 3 minutes   **COOK TIME:** 20 minutes
PER SERVING: *calories 301; fat 5 g; saturated fat 2 g; fiber 4.5 g; protein 11 g; carbohydrates 54 g; sugar 9.5 g*

1 large French baguette
1½ cups Marinara Sauce (page 103)
1½ cups shredded mozzarella cheese

OPTIONAL TOPPINGS
Diced bell pepper
Diced onion
Sliced mushrooms
Sliced olives
Diced pineapple
Minced or sliced jalapeños
Halved artichoke hearts
Nitrate-free pepperoni

1. Preheat the oven to 375°F.

2. Slice the bread lengthwise in thirds, to get three very long, thin slices. Place the bread on a sheet pan. Top evenly with the marinara sauce, mozzarella, and any desired toppings.

3. Bake for 15 to 20 minutes, until the cheese has melted and the bread is crispy and golden along the edges.

4. Let the pizzas cool for 5 minutes, then cut each in half and serve.

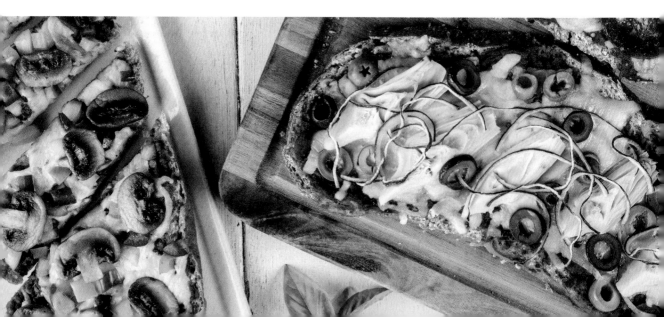

Marinara Sauce

It just wouldn't be a Lose Weight by Eating cookbook without a marinara recipe. In this versatile version I supply three easy ways to cook it, so you can pick the method that's most convenient for you.

With this recipe, you can make several fast dinners throughout the week! Try French Bread Pizzas (page 102) for a quick weeknight meal.

○ **SERVING SIZE:** 1 cup **PREP TIME:** 3 minutes
COOK TIME: 4 hours for stovetop and slow cooker, 30 minutes for the Instant Pot
PER SERVING: *calories 135; fat 1.5 g; saturated fat 0 g; fiber 8.5 g; protein 7 g; carbohydrates 27 g; sugar 18 g*

1 teaspoon olive oil
1 medium yellow onion, minced
5 garlic cloves, minced
⅓ cup chopped fresh basil leaves
1 (28-ounce) can crushed tomatoes
1 (15-ounce) can tomato sauce
1 (6-ounce) can tomato paste
½ teaspoon sugar
Pinch of kosher salt
Pinch of freshly ground black pepper

STOVETOP INSTRUCTIONS

1. In a large saucepan, heat the oil over medium-low heat. Add the onion and sauté for 5 minutes, or until the onion is soft. Add the garlic and cook for 2 minutes, until fragrant.

2. Add the basil, crushed tomatoes, tomato sauce, tomato paste, 1 cup water, the sugar, and the salt. Cook over low heat for 4 to 8 hours, stirring every 30 minutes to avoid burning.

INSTANT POT INSTRUCTIONS

1. Combine the oil and onion in an Instant Pot. Set the pot to sauté on medium heat and cook for 5 minutes, or until the onion is soft. Add the garlic and cook for 2 minutes, until fragrant. Hit cancel.

2. Add the basil, crushed tomatoes, tomato sauce, tomato paste, 1 cup water, the sugar, and the salt to the pot, cover, and cook on high pressure for 30 minutes. Let the pressure release naturally.

SLOW COOKER INSTRUCTIONS

1. In a large skillet, heat the oil over medium-low heat. Add the onion and sauté for 5 minutes, or until the onion is soft. Add the garlic and cook for 2 minutes, until fragrant.

2. Transfer the onion and garlic to a slow cooker and add the basil, crushed tomatoes, tomato sauce, tomato paste, 1 cup water, the sugar, and the salt. Cover and cook on high for 4 hours or low for 8 to 12 hours.

LEFTOVERS TIPS: I like to freeze leftover sauce in a gallon freezer bag. Lay it flat to freeze, then once it's solid you can fit it in even the most packed freezer. Alternatively, you can store the sauce for up to 1 week in the fridge in a glass container: I like mason jars.

MIX-AND-MATCH PROTEINS AND SIDE DISHES

This mix-and-match chapter makes meal planning easy! Just pick a protein and a side and you're done.

But don't stop there with the mixing and matching. . . . Is it a hot summer afternoon? Skip the side dish and make a filling salad from chapter 2 instead. Is it a chilly winter night? Choose a soup from chapter 2 in place of a side or main dish.

PROTEINS

SIDE DISHES

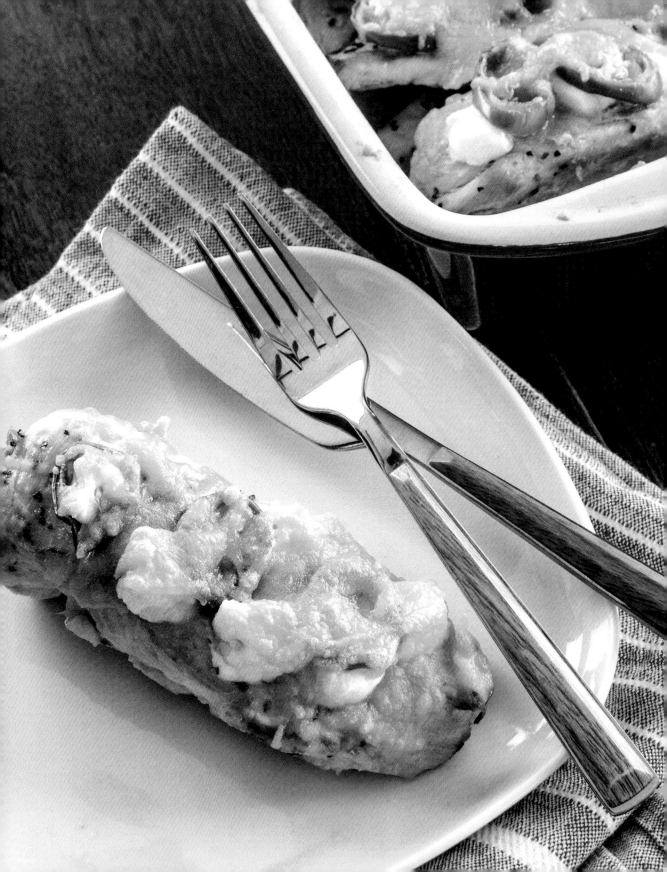

Jalapeño Popper Chicken

🥞 **MAKES 4 SERVINGS**

This can be made mild, medium, or hot, depending on how you cut your peppers. Here's how:

- **MILD:** Remove all the ribs and seeds from the jalapeño.
- **MEDIUM:** Remove all the seeds and leave the ribs.
- **HOT:** Leave it as is . . . or add more jalapeño slices to make it *really* hot.

SERVING SIZE: 1 chicken breast   **PREP TIME:** 2 minutes   **COOK TIME:** 25 minutes
PER SERVING: *calories 416; fat 18 g; saturated fat 6.5 g; fiber 0 g; protein 58 g; carbohydrates 0 g; sugar 0 g*

Olive oil spray
4 (4-ounce) boneless, skinless chicken breasts
Kosher salt and freshly ground black pepper
4 teaspoons light cream cheese (Neufchâtel cheese)
1 jalapeño, sliced
⅓ cup shredded cheddar cheese

1. Preheat the oven to 450°F. Lightly spray a sheet pan with olive oil.

2. Lay the chicken on the sheet pan and lightly sprinkle it with salt and pepper. Top each breast with 1 teaspoon of the cream cheese, some jalapeño, and a sprinkling of the cheddar.

3. Bake for 20 to 25 minutes, until the chicken is cooked through. Serve hot. I like this chicken with a crisp salad.

Pizza Chicken Breasts

Okay, I know what you're thinking . . . this can't be healthy. But it is, *if* you're smart with your ingredients. First of all, get the good, nitrate-free pepperoni . . . yes, it's more expensive ($3 vs. $1.50 for the other stuff), but you use only a little and you can freeze the rest! Second . . . do you notice the lack of dough/bread? I'll wait while you look at the ingredients. . . .

You can curb your cravings with healthy meals like this one that approximate the flavors of less-healthy foods you love. I recommend pairing this with Kale Caesar Salad (page 26).

◎ **SERVING SIZE:** 1 chicken breast　**PREP TIME:** 10 minutes　**COOK TIME:** 30 minutes
　PER SERVING: *calories 421; fat 19 g; saturated fat 5.5 g; fiber 0.5 g; protein 57 g; carbohydrates 2 g; sugar 2 g*

---

4 (4-ounce) boneless, skinless chicken breasts
Kosher salt and freshly ground black pepper
2 garlic cloves, grated
¾ cup tomato sauce
½ cup shredded mozzarella cheese
8 slices nitrate-free pepperoni, quartered

1. Preheat the oven to 450°F.

2. Place a 3-foot piece of plastic wrap on a cutting board and lay one chicken breast in the center of the wrap. Fold the plastic wrap over so that the chicken is covered and use the flat side of a meat tenderizer (or a rolling pin) to bash it until it's flattened to ⅛ inch thick. Repeat with the remaining breasts. As you finish each piece, sprinkle it with salt and pepper and place it in a single layer in a 9 × 13-inch baking pan.

3. In a medium bowl, combine the garlic, tomato sauce, and a pinch each of salt and pepper.

4. Top each chicken breast evenly with the tomato sauce mixture, the mozzarella, and the pepperoni.

5. Bake for 20 to 25 minutes, until the chicken is cooked through and the cheese is melted. Switch the oven to broil and cook for another 2 to 5 minutes to brown the cheese. Serve hot.

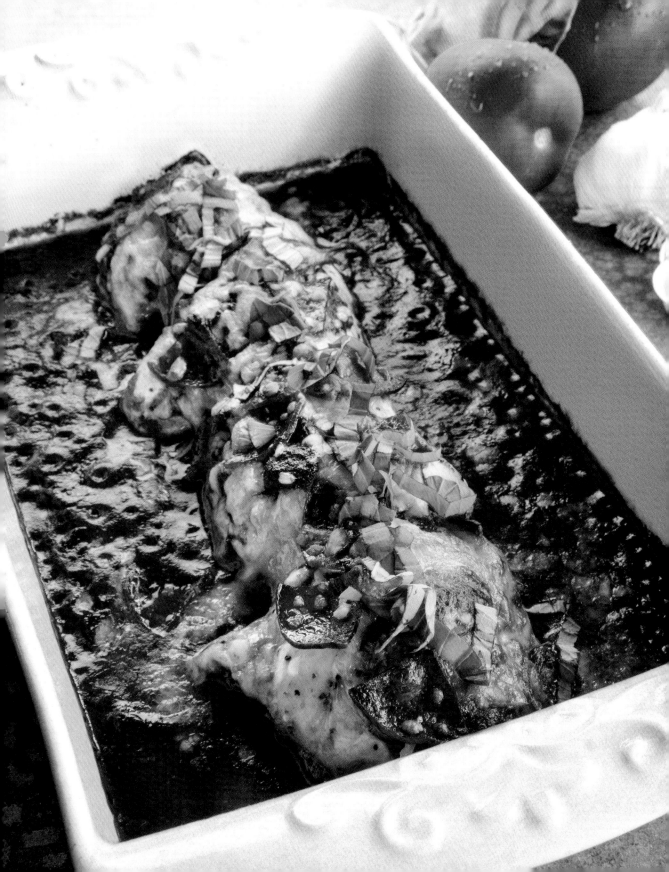

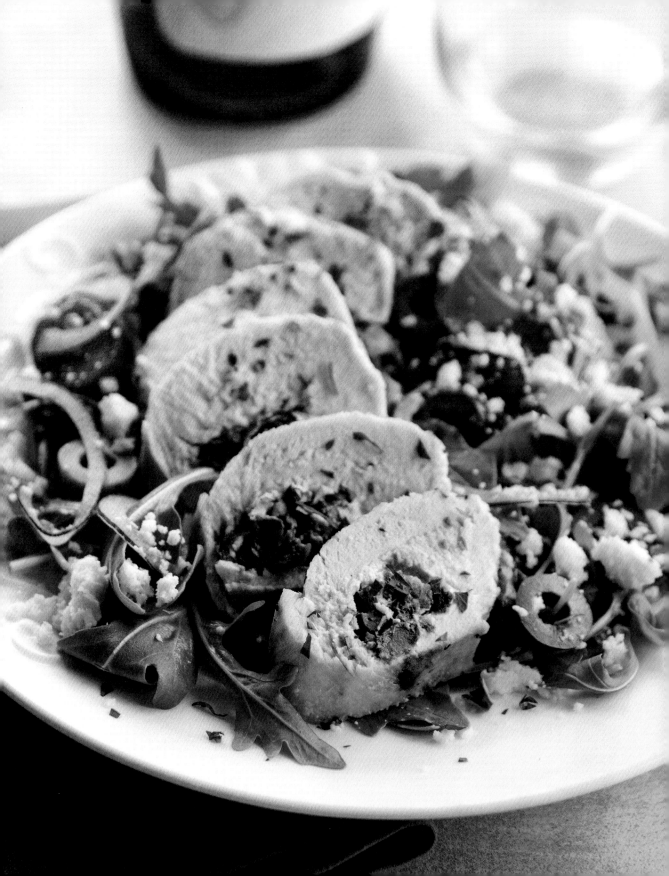

Mediterranean Stuffed Chicken

🍥 **MAKES 2 SERVINGS**

This combination of ingredients makes up one of my favorite flavor profiles . . . and it's so flexible when it comes to substitutions. Feel free to use feta cheese in place of the goat cheese, or sliced peperoncini in place of the olives, for example. And having these basic pantry ingredients stocked means you can make lots of delicious dishes from this and my other cookbooks. In this book alone, they'll help you make Simple Greek Salad (page 21), Hummus Bowl (page 93), and Greek Chicken and Rice (page 84).

◯ **SERVING SIZE:** 1 chicken breast and ½ cup greens   **PREP TIME:** 5 minutes   **COOK TIME:** 20 minutes
PER SERVING: *calories 395; fat 18 g; saturated fat 6 g; fiber 0.5 g; protein 54 g; carbohydrates 2 g; sugar 0 g*

2 (4-ounce) boneless, skinless chicken breasts
2 tablespoons crumbled goat cheese
2 tablespoons minced sun-dried tomatoes
2 tablespoons sliced Kalamata olives
Kosher salt and freshly ground black pepper
Olive oil spray
1 cup mixed greens

1. Preheat the oven to 425°F.

2. Place a chicken breast on a cutting board and, using a small sharp knife, slice horizontally into the fatter side of the breast and continue cutting to make a pocket inside. (Place your hand on the top of the chicken breast as you cut through to steady it.) Repeat with the second breast.

3. Stuff the pockets in the chicken breasts with the goat cheese, sun-dried tomatoes, and olives, dividing them evenly. Close them up and lightly sprinkle with salt and pepper. Lightly spray with olive oil and place in a baking dish.

4. Bake for 20 to 25 minutes, until cooked through and browned. Serve the chicken over the mixed greens or your favorite Mediterranean salad.

Lemon Pepper Grilled Chicken

🥫 **MAKES 4 SERVINGS**

My special guy and I frequent a hole-in-the-wall restaurant that makes the best chicken and saffron rice. This amazing little family-owned restaurant inspired this dish, and I pride myself on the fact that it is very close to their version. This goes amazingly well with Saffron Rice (page 114) and Simple Greek Salad (page 21).

I made this for two, but it can easily be scaled up for four, six, eight, or more. And the chicken makes wonderful leftovers for salads!

◎ **SERVING SIZE:** 1 chicken cutlet   **PREP TIME:** 3 minutes   **COOK TIME:** 15 minutes
PER SERVING: *calories 207; fat 2.5 g; saturated fat 0 g; fiber 0 g; protein 43 g; carbohydrates 2 g; sugar 2 g*

---

2 (4-ounce) boneless, skinless chicken breasts
Grated zest and juice of 1 lemon
½ cup 0% Greek yogurt
2 garlic cloves, grated
1 teaspoon freshly ground black pepper
¼ teaspoon kosher salt

1. Place a chicken breast on a cutting board and, using a small sharp knife, slice horizontally into the fatter side of the breast and cut all the way through to make 2 thin cutlets. (Place your hand on the top of the chicken breast as you cut through to steady it.) Repeat with the second breast.

2. Add the lemon zest, lemon juice, yogurt, garlic, salt, pepper, and 2 tablespoons water to a gallon freezer bag. Add the chicken, seal the bag, and squish the bag to mix everything, then place the bag in a baking dish. Marinate in the fridge for at least 2 hours and up to 24 hours. Flip and squish every so often . . . basically whenever you remember to.

3. Preheat a grill to high heat.

4. Remove the chicken from the marinade (discard the marinade). Grill, covered, for 5 to 8 minutes on each side, until cooked through. Serve hot.

Spanish Rice and Beans

This is one of those foolproof side dishes that even picky eaters love. Part of it is the simplicity of the ingredients, and part of it is the topping bar you can offer. Everyone loves a dish they can personalize.

SERVING SIZE: ½ cup   **PREP TIME:** 5 minutes   **COOK TIME:** 30 minutes
PER SERVING: *calories 300; fat 2.5 g; saturated fat 0.5 g; fiber 11 g; protein 16 g; carbohydrates 54 g; sugar 4 g*

1½ teaspoons olive oil
1 medium yellow onion, minced
Pinch of kosher salt
Pinch of freshly ground black pepper
2 garlic cloves, minced
½ cup long-grain white rice
1 (14.5-ounce) can diced tomatoes
1 cup low-sodium chicken broth or vegetable broth
1 teaspoon chili powder
1 (15.5-ounce) can pinto beans, drained and rinsed

OPTIONAL TOPPINGS
Chopped fresh cilantro
Shredded cheddar cheese
0% Greek yogurt (in place of sour cream)
Salsa
Sliced green onions
Crushed tortilla chips

1. In a medium saucepan, heat the oil over medium-low heat. Add the onion, salt, and pepper. Sauté for 5 minutes, until the onion is softened. Add the garlic and sauté for 1 minute, until fragrant.

2. Add the rice and cook for 3 minutes, stirring often. Add the tomatoes, broth, and chili powder. Cover and bring to a boil over medium-high heat. Reduce the heat to low and cook until all the liquid is absorbed, 15 to 20 minutes.

3. Fluff with a fork, add the beans, and mix to combine. Serve with your desired toppings.

Once-a-Week Cooking

Saffron Rice

I almost always have some leftover saffron rice in my fridge. After I created this recipe, I became obsessed with it! It's great as a side dish, but I also like to add it to my salads the next day.

I know what you're thinking . . . saffron is expensive, and yes, for a spice it is. But you use such a small amount in this recipe that it will last you a long time, so technically it's an investment ingredient. Trust me on this—it's well worth the price!

○ **SERVING SIZE:** ½ cup   **PREP TIME:** 2 minutes   **COOK TIME:** 20 minutes
  PER SERVING: *calories 169; fat 0.5 g; saturated fat 0 g; fiber 0.5 g; protein 3 g; carbohydrates 37 g; sugar 0 g*

⅛ teaspoon (1 pinch) saffron threads
¼ cup boiling water
1 cup long-grain white rice
½ teaspoon ground cumin
½ teaspoon garlic powder
½ teaspoon onion powder
Kosher salt and freshly ground black pepper

1. In a medium saucepan, combine the saffron and boiling water and let sit, covered, for at least 30 minutes (or all day if you like).

2. Add the rice, cumin, garlic powder, onion powder, and a pinch each of salt and pepper to the pan. Add 1¾ cups water and mix to combine. Cover and cook over low heat until all the water is absorbed, 15 to 20 minutes.

3. Fluff with a fork. Season with salt to taste and serve.

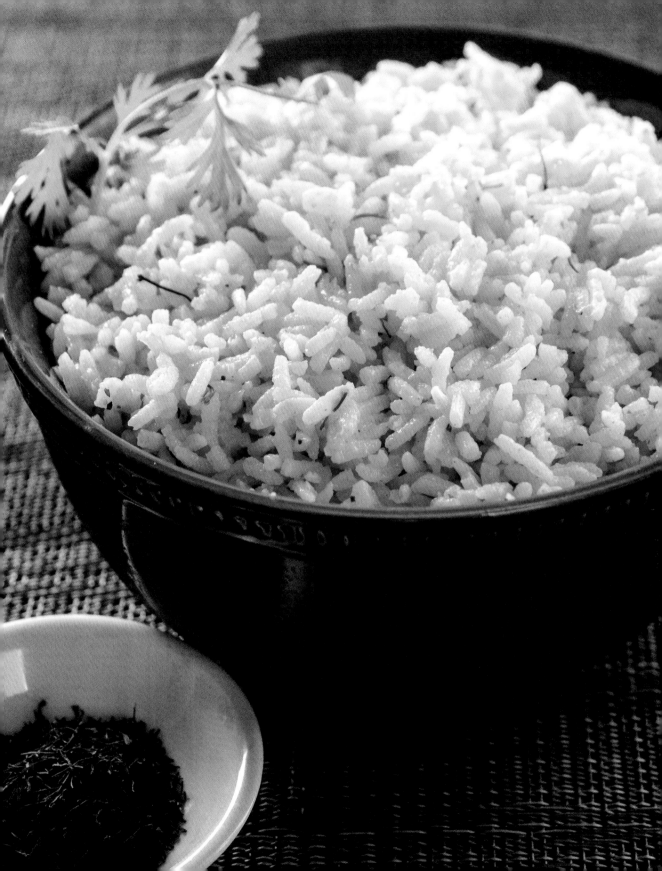

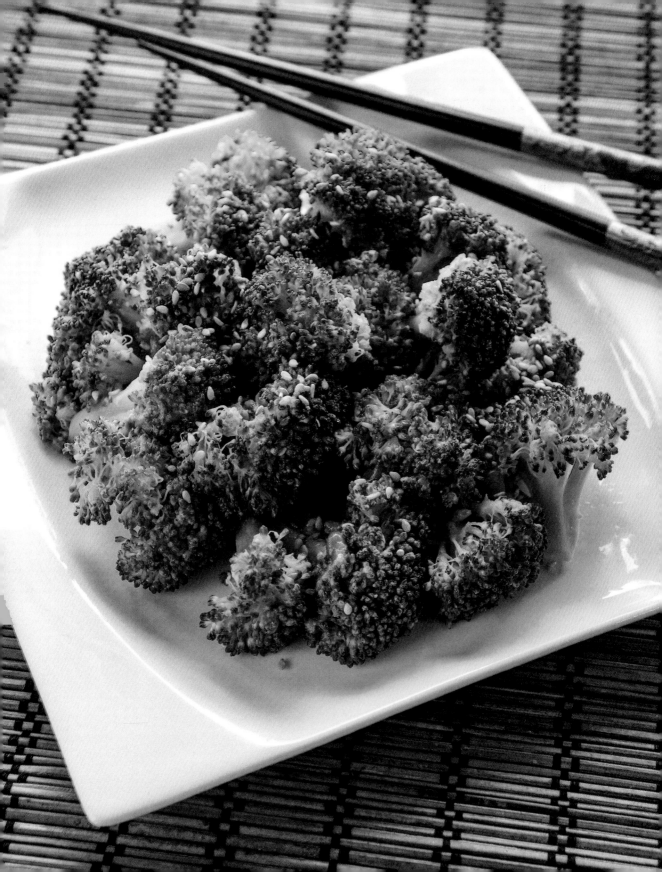

Miso-Sesame Broccoli

MAKES 2 SERVINGS

I purchased some gluten-free miso paste online, and now I feel compelled to cook with it whenever my special guy comes over. This is what drove the creation of this recipe, and I make this often with both regular miso paste and the gluten-free version, depending on who I'm cooking for.

SERVING SIZE: 1 cup   **PREP TIME:** 5 minutes   **COOK TIME:** 20 minutes
PER SERVING: *calories 83; fat 4 g; saturated fat 0.5 g; fiber 3 g; protein 4 g; carbohydrates 9 g; sugar 2 g*

---

2 cups broccoli florets
1 teaspoon toasted sesame oil
1 tablespoon miso paste
1½ teaspoons soy sauce (or tamari, for a gluten-free meal)
1½ teaspoons sesame seeds

1. Preheat the oven to 450°F.

2. Spread the broccoli in a 9 × 13-inch baking dish. In a small bowl, combine the sesame oil, miso, and soy sauce. Pour over the broccoli, toss to combine, and top with the sesame seeds.

3. Bake for 20 minutes, or until tender, mixing halfway through. Serve hot.

Sweet or Savory Hasselback Sweet Potatoes

🍥 **MAKES 1 SERVING**

I wasn't sure if I wanted this to be a sweet or a savory recipe, so I tested both . . . and, well, I still can't decide which one is better, so I kept them both. The sweet version is great with pork chops and the savory is fantastic with roast chicken. Or do as I did—make both and enjoy a half portion of each version.

This is a one-serving recipe, so if you have more to feed, just increase the ingredients accordingly. The bake time will be the same regardless.

◎ **SERVING SIZE:** 1 sweet potato   **PREP TIME:** 5 minutes   **COOK TIME:** 50 minutes
PER SERVING: *calories 114; fat 0 g; saturated fat 0 g; fiber 4 g; protein 2 g; carbohydrates 26 g; sugar 10 g*

---

1 medium sweet potato (about 4 ounces), scrubbed
Olive oil spray

SWEET TOPPINGS
1 teaspoon light brown sugar
¼ teaspoon pumpkin pie spice
⅛ teaspoon kosher salt

SAVORY TOPPINGS
1 (2-inch) fresh rosemary sprig
1 teaspoon freshly grated Parmesan cheese
⅛ teaspoon kosher salt
⅛ teaspoon freshly ground black pepper

1. Preheat the oven to 425°F. Line a sheet pan with foil or parchment paper.

2. Slice the sweet potato Hasselback style. The easiest way to do this is to place the potato in a wooden spoon (it won't quite fit, but you can move it as you work) so that the spoon cradles the bottom of the potato. You can then slice down to the edge of the spoon without cutting all the way through.

3. Place the sweet potato on the baking sheet, lightly spray it with olive oil, and bake for 35 minutes.

4. Add the sweet or savory toppings and bake for 15 minutes more, until tender in the center. Discard the rosemary sprig, or use it as a garnish. Serve hot.

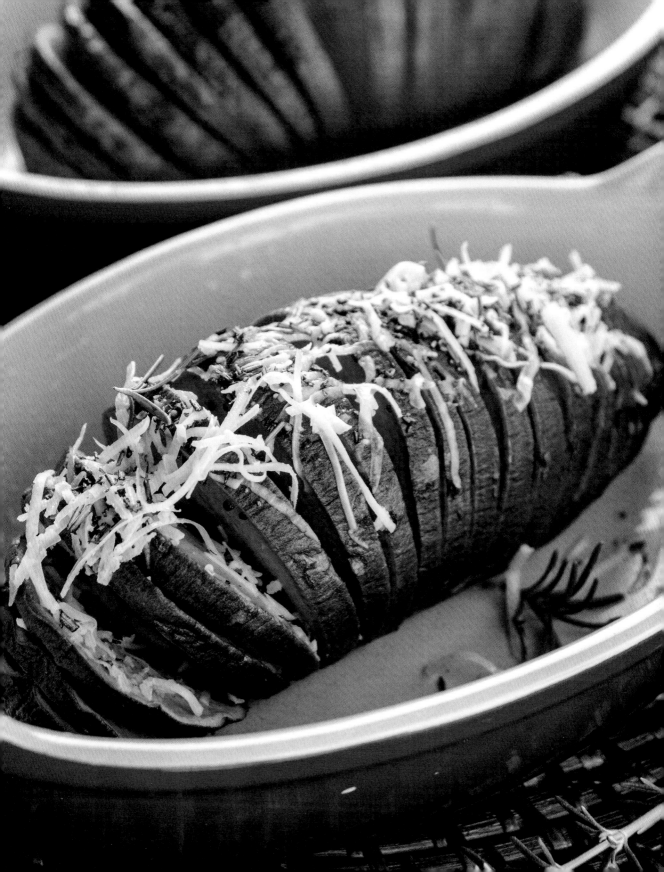

Mashed Sweet Potatoes

For those of you looking for a new "mashed potato" recipe, try out this sweet potato version.

Now, I love potatoes . . . like, a lot! But I've been trying to work more sweet potatoes into my diet. They have fewer calories and more fiber and won't spike your blood sugar levels as much. I chose vegan butter to include more recipes for vegan readers. You can use whatever butter you have on hand.

SERVING SIZE: about ⅔ cup **PREP TIME:** 8 minutes **COOK TIME:** 25 minutes
PER SERVING: *calories 136; fat 2 g; saturated fat 1.5 g; fiber 4 g; protein 1 g; carbohydrates 28 g; sugar 0.5 g*

---

1 tablespoon kosher salt, plus more to taste
2 large sweet potatoes (about 6 ounces each)
2 garlic cloves
2 tablespoons vegan or regular butter, cut into small cubes
2 teaspoons chili powder
Freshly ground black pepper

1. Fill a large saucepan two-thirds full of water, add the salt, and set the pan next to your cutting board. Peel the sweet potatoes and cut them into 1-inch chunks, placing them in the water as you work.

2. Add the garlic cloves to the pan and bring to a boil over medium-high heat. Cook for 15 to 25 minutes, until the sweet potato chunks are soft in the center when poked with a fork. Drain the water.

3. Use a potato masher to smash the sweet potatoes with half the butter until smooth. Add salt and pepper to taste, transfer to a 9 × 9-inch casserole dish, drop the remaining butter cubes evenly over the top, and serve immediately. You can also cover with foil and reheat in a 350°F oven for 20 minutes.

Twice-Baked Mexican Sweet Potatoes

🥞 **MAKES 2 SERVINGS**

This recipe makes a great meal as well as a side dish. To make it a meal, simply add ½ cup shredded cooked chicken to the stuffing (if you're not into meat, add some avocado slices before serving instead) and eat the whole potato instead of half.

I've been having a bit of a love affair with sweet potatoes for quite some time now; I'm always looking for new ways to cook with them. They are so nutritious and inexpensive (even when buying organic), so I always pick up a few when I grocery shop. If you prefer russet or golden potatoes to sweet potatoes, by all means, swap them in—this recipe is delicious with savory potatoes, too!

◯ **SERVING SIZE:** ½ potato   **PREP TIME:** 3 minutes   **COOK TIME:** 20 minutes
PER SERVING: *calories 140; fat 6.5 g; saturated fat 4 g; fiber 2.5 g; protein 6 g; carbohydrates 15 g; sugar 4.5 g*

---

1 medium sweet potato (about 4 ounces)
1 green onion, thinly sliced
1 jalapeño, diced (seeds and ribs removed for a milder dish)
2 tablespoons frozen corn kernels
⅓ cup shredded sharp cheddar cheese
½ teaspoon ground cumin
½ teaspoon garlic powder
½ teaspoon chili powder
Kosher salt and freshly ground black pepper

1. Preheat the oven to 425°F.

2. Stab the sweet potato a few times with a fork, then bake for 1 hour, until it is tender when you squeeze it gently. (Alternatively, microwave the sweet potato for 5 minutes).

3. Let the sweet potato cool for a few minutes or use oven mitts to handle it (you'll probably want to do both). Halve the potato lengthwise, then use a spoon to scoop out about two-thirds of the inside flesh and transfer it to a medium bowl, reserving the skins, which will now resemble canoes.

4. Add the green onion, jalapeño, corn, half the cheddar, the cumin, garlic powder, and chili powder to the bowl with the sweet potato and mix well. Season with salt and black pepper to taste.

5. Spoon the stuffing into the potato skins, top with the remaining cheese, and place on a sheet pan. Bake for 15 minutes, until the cheese is melted and bubbling. Serve hot.

AFTER DINNER

A Lose Weight by Eating cookbook wouldn't be complete without a dessert chapter!

I like to make a batch of Frozen Chocolate Cherries (page 126) and Peanut Butter Bites (page 125) at the same time. I figure I'm already dealing with melted chocolate and the freezer. This ensures I'm well stocked on low-calorie, high-nutrition treats for days (or weeks, depending on my stress levels).

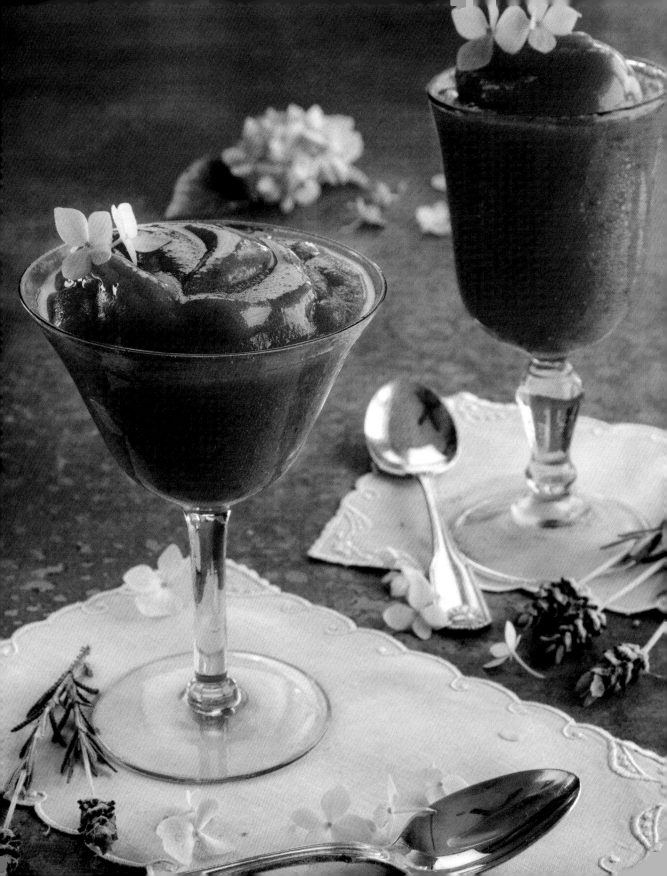

Strawberry Rosé Granita

🎂 **MAKES 6 SERVINGS**

This boozy treat can be made nonalcoholic easily. Swap out the wine and the honey for ½ cup all-natural lemon-lime soda. Easy and great for everyone in the family. To make this a vegan dessert, simply swap out the honey and replace it with agave or your favorite all-natural liquid sweetener.

⚪ **SERVING SIZE:** ½ cup **PREP TIME:** 2 minutes **COOK TIME:** 0 minutes
PER SERVING: *calories 43; fat 0 g; saturated fat 0 g; fiber 0.5 g; protein 0 g; carbohydrates 8 g; sugar 7 g*

---

1 cup whole strawberries (frozen or fresh)
1 cup rosé wine
2 tablespoons honey

1. In a blender, combine all the ingredients and blend until smooth.

2. Pour into a freezer-safe container and place in the freezer for 3 hours. Every hour, remove the mixture and scrape/break it up with a fork, then return it to the freezer. This keeps your granita from turning into one large ice cube.

3. Serve in a pretty glass to your of-age friends.

Peanut Butter Banana Bites

🎂 **MAKES 10 SERVINGS**

My daughter and I fight over these. . . . No joke, we race to the freezer to get the best ones and we fight over who gets the last one. Get vegan chocolate chips to make this recipe vegan.

⚪ **SERVING SIZE:** 2 **PREP TIME:** 5 minutes **COOK TIME:** 1 minute
PER SERVING: *calories 49; fat 3 g; saturated fat 1.5 g; fiber 0.5 g; protein 1 g; carbohydrates 6 g; sugar 3.5 g*

---

1 large banana, cut into ¼-inch-thick slices (about 20 slices)
2 tablespoons peanut butter (crunchy or creamy, whatever you prefer)
¼ cup dark chocolate chips
1 teaspoon coconut oil

1. Line a plate with parchment paper. Arrange the banana slices on the plate (not touching). Spoon a small amount of peanut butter on top of each banana slice.

2. In a microwave-safe bowl, combine the chocolate chips and coconut oil. Microwave in 10-second increments, mixing after each, until completely melted.

3. Spoon the chocolate over the peanut butter–covered bananas. Make room in your freezer for the plate and freeze the bananas for 1 hour to set before enjoying.

4. Store in the freezer. You can move them from the plate to a freezer bag for storage once completely frozen.

After Dinner

Frozen Chocolate Cherries

🥫 **MAKES 8 SERVINGS**

The hardest part of this recipe (which honestly isn't difficult at all) is melting the chocolate. So, I double the chocolate and make lots of treats. They all stay in the freezer, so why not, right?!

One note here: Unless you have a cherry tree and you're desperately looking for ways to use up your harvest, get frozen cherries. Have you ever pitted a ton of cherries? Your kitchen will look like a crime scene! So, save your clothing and the time it would take cleaning blood-red cherry juice off your countertops and use frozen pitted cherries. . . plus, you'll likely save a lot of money. Get vegan chocolate chips to make this recipe vegan.

◎ **SERVING SIZE:** 2 cherries   **PREP TIME:** 2 minutes   **COOK TIME:** 1 minute
PER SERVING: *calories 32; fat 1.5 g; saturated fat 1 g; fiber 0.5 g; protein 0 g; carbohydrates 5 g; sugar 4 g*

---

16 frozen pitted red cherries
¼ cup dark chocolate chips
1 teaspoon coconut oil

1. Line a plate with parchment paper. Place the cherries on the plate (not touching).

2. In a microwave-safe bowl, combine the chocolate chips and coconut oil. Microwave in 10-second increments, mixing after each, until completely melted.

3. Spoon the chocolate over the cherries. Clear a space in your freezer for the plate and freeze the cherries for 1 hour to set before digging in.

4. Store in the freezer. You can move them from the plate to a freezer bag for storage once completely frozen.

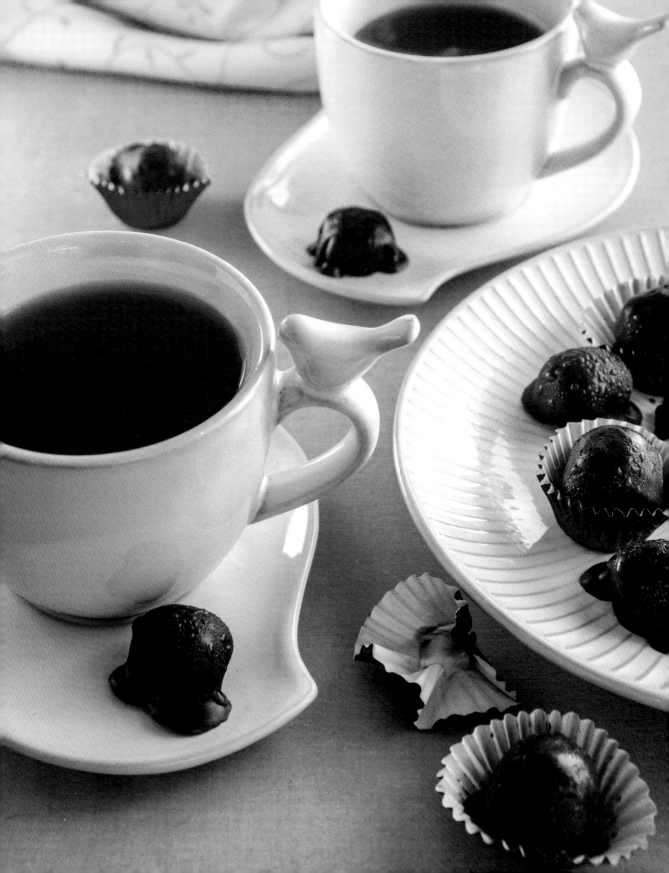

Baked Blueberry Apples

These are not only delicious and impressive, but they also make your house smell heavenly!

I like to split one of these apples with someone as a dessert, as a whole one is very filling. These apples also make amazing breakfasts, and at 226 calories, they have just enough calories to get your metabolism jump-started in the morning.

SERVING SIZE: 1 apple   **PREP TIME:** 5 minutes   **COOK TIME:** 1 hour
PER SERVING: *calories 226; fat 4.5 g; saturated fat 3 g; fiber 7.5 g; protein 3 g; carbohydrates 47 g; sugar 3 g*

---

2 apples (sweet varieties are best)
¼ cup fresh or frozen blueberries
1 tablespoon dark brown sugar
2 tablespoons old-fashioned rolled oats
1½ teaspoons coconut oil

1. Preheat the oven to 350°F.

2. Core the apples partway from the top down, removing the core and seeds but leaving the bottom intact. I like to use a paring knife to cut a circle around the core, then scoop it out with a spoon.

3. Place the apples in a baking dish and fill the wells with the blueberries.

4. In a small bowl, combine the brown sugar, oats, and coconut oil. Sprinkle the mixture over the tops of the apples.

5. Bake for 1 hour, or until the apples are soft and the topping is browned. (I like to put these in the oven to bake while we eat dinner.)

6. Let sit for 10 minutes before serving or they will be blazing hot in the center.

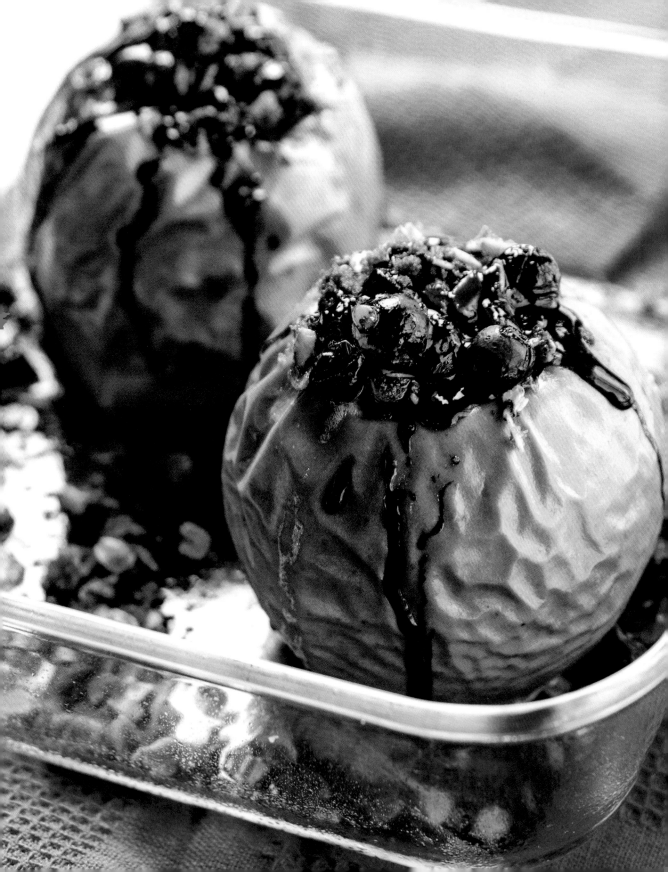

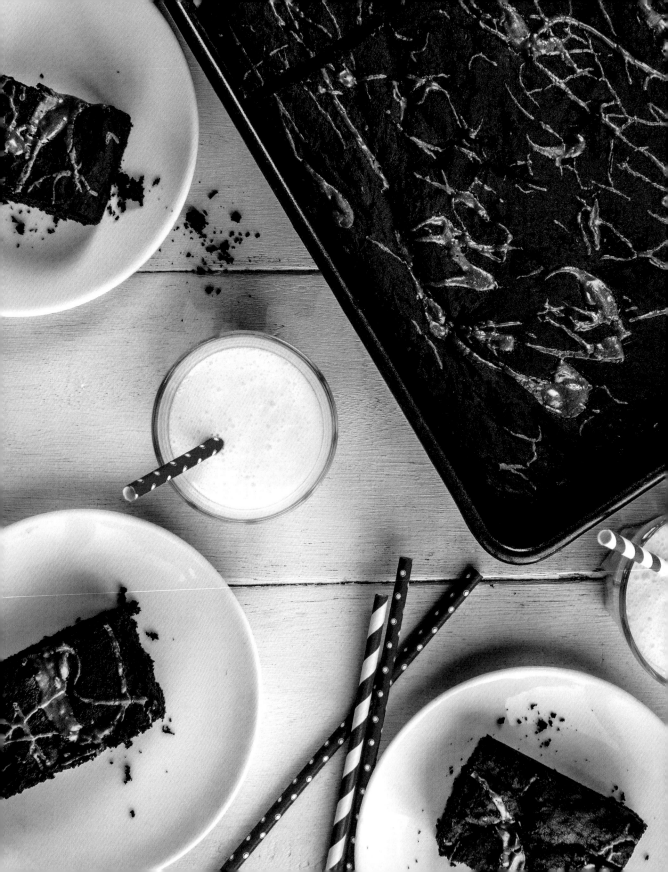

Gluten-Free Peanut Butter Brownies

🍪 **MAKES 21 BROWNIES**

The first time I made this recipe, I made it two ways. The first batch was made with traditional all-purpose flour, and the second batch I made with gluten-free baking flour. I was pleased to find that the gluten-free brownies were just as good, if not slightly better, than the wheat flour brownies.

Gluten-free all-purpose flour is more expensive than traditional all-purpose flour and the quality difference isn't drastic, so by all means use what you have on hand if gluten isn't a concern.

◯ **SERVING SIZE:** 1 brownie   **PREP TIME:** 2 minutes   **COOK TIME:** 20 minutes
PER SERVING: *calories 155; fat 6.5 g; saturated fat 4 g; fiber 1 g; protein 9 g; carbohydrates 17 g; sugar 11 g*

¼ cup coconut oil, plus more for the pan
1 cup dark chocolate chips
½ cup coconut sugar or packed light
   brown sugar
1 cup 0% Greek yogurt
1 teaspoon pure vanilla extract
2 large eggs
½ cup unsweetened cocoa powder
1 heaping teaspoon baking soda
1¼ cups Bob's Red Mill Gluten-Free 1-to-1
   Baking Flour
½ teaspoon kosher salt
¼ cup creamy peanut butter

1. Preheat the oven to 350°F. Lightly oil a 9 × 13-inch baking dish with coconut oil.

2. In a large saucepan, melt the coconut oil, chocolate chips, and coconut sugar over medium-low heat, stirring until smooth and well combined. Remove from the heat and set aside to cool for about 5 minutes.

3. Whisk in the yogurt and vanilla. At this point the mixture should be at room temperature; if not, let it sit for another

5 minutes. Whisk in the eggs until combined. Whisk in the cocoa powder, baking soda, flour, and salt until you have a smooth, mousse-like batter.

4. Scrape the batter into the prepared baking dish and smooth it to the edges in an even layer.

5. In a microwave-safe bowl, microwave the peanut butter in 15-second increments, stirring after each, until it's very smooth and runny. Drizzle the peanut butter over the brownie batter, letting it drip and splatter in a very Jackson Pollock fashion.

6. Bake for 15 to 20 minutes, until the outer one-third of the brownies is firm to the touch.

7. Let the brownies cool completely in the baking dish; they will continue to firm up as they cool. Slice the brownies into 21 brownie bars (two long cuts and six short cuts). Cover and store in the fridge for up to 5 days.

MARINADES, SAUCES, AND RUBS ... OH MY!

D inner can be challenging at times! I hope this cookbook has supplied you with easy dinner recipes to remove some of the difficulty.

I want to leave you with a quick "one stop" chapter for those nights when you don't want to follow a recipe. Or for afternoons when you have gone grocery shopping, found chicken on sale, and need a marinade. The following recipes will both assist you in completing dinner recipes within this book, and hopefully inspire you to create some new ones yourself.

Citrus Marinade

🥫 **MAKES ABOUT 1 CUP**

This marinade is great on chicken, tofu, and fish. On the grill, in the pan, and even in the oven.

Juice of 3 oranges or 3 lemons, or a combo of both (I like 2 oranges and 1 lemon)
5 garlic cloves, grated
1½ teaspoons kosher salt
3 fresh thyme sprigs

1. In a medium bowl, whisk together the citrus juice, garlic, and salt.

2. Pour the marinade over the protein of your choice, or into a bag with the protein, and top with the thyme.

FOR CHICKEN: Marinate for 1 to 24 hours—the longer the better!

FOR TOFU: Marinate for 2 to 6 hours.

FOR FISH OR SHRIMP: Marinate for 15 to 20 minutes.

Taco Marinade

🥫 **MAKES ABOUT ¼ CUP**

I use this marinade for shredded chicken tacos, but you can also make ground meat tacos, crumbled tofu tacos, or even fajitas with this one.

Juice of 1 lime
1 garlic clove, minced
1 teaspoon chili powder
½ teaspoon ground cumin
¼ teaspoon Italian seasoning

1. In a small bowl or zip-top bag, combine all the ingredients.

2. There are two ways to use this marinade:

- Marinate meat (such as chicken) in the fridge for up to 12 hours.

- Brown ground beef or turkey or crumbled tofu for tacos, and add the marinade with 2 tablespoons water.

Garlic Pesto Sauce

🥫 **MAKES ABOUT ½ CUP**

Mix this with 0% Greek yogurt for a flavorful sandwich spread, or toss a few tablespoons in a bowl of pasta for a quick dinner. It goes great over chicken and even veggies.

2 cups fresh basil leaves
2 teaspoons extra-virgin or regular olive oil
2 tablespoons freshly grated Parmesan cheese
4 garlic cloves

In a blender or food processor, combine all the ingredients and process until mostly smooth, adding water 1 teaspoon at a time to thin it to the desired consistency. It will keep in an airtight container for 2 or 3 days in the fridge.

Korean Barbecue Sauce

🥫 **MAKES ABOUT 1 CUP**

This sweet and spicy sauce goes great over beef and chicken, into shredded pork, over veggies . . . you'll want to use it everywhere.

1 (4-ounce) jar pear baby food
¼ cup packed dark brown sugar
¼ cup soy sauce (or tamari, for a gluten-free sauce)
1 tablespoon rice vinegar
½ to 1 tablespoon chili garlic paste (depending on how hot you like it)
1 teaspoon toasted sesame oil
1 teaspoon grated fresh ginger
Pinch of freshly ground black pepper

1. In a small saucepan, combine the pear baby food, brown sugar, soy sauce, vinegar, chili garlic paste, sesame oil, ginger, pepper, and ¼ cup water. Bring to a boil over medium-low heat. Reduce the heat to maintain a simmer and cook for 5 minutes, until thickened.

2. Cool in the fridge. The sauce will keep in an airtight container in the fridge for 1 week.

Buffalo Sauce

MAKES ABOUT 1 CUP

The secret to this Buffalo sauce is Frank's RedHot. It's both spicy and vinegary, perfect for Buffalo sauce.

1 cup Frank's RedHot sauce
¼ cup fresh lemon juice
2 teaspoons garlic salt
2 teaspoons paprika
1 teaspoon cayenne pepper
1 teaspoon freshly ground black pepper

In a small bowl, combine all the ingredients. Cover and store in the fridge for up to 1 week.

Cayenne Rub

MAKES ABOUT 3 TABLESPOONS

I love using rubs; they add zero calories but lots of flavor. This is my favorite steak rub and—don't fret—it's not too spicy! But if you're concerned about the heat, you can cut the cayenne in half. Rub it on steaks or other protein.

1 tablespoon garlic powder
1 tablespoon paprika
1 teaspoon ground cumin
½ teaspoon cayenne pepper
¼ teaspoon kosher salt
¼ teaspoon freshly ground black pepper

In a small bowl, mix together all the ingredients. Store in a sealed container in your pantry for up to 3 months.

Ranch Dressing Rub

I keep coming across recipes that call for a packet of dry ranch mix, but all the preservatives in the store-bought mixture are detrimental to your health and weight loss goals. So, I made this ranch rub recipe for all of you.

You can use it as a traditional rub—it's amazing on chicken before grilling—or you can use it in place of the store-bought stuff. You can even add some 0% Greek yogurt and turn it into a dip or marinade.

1 tablespoon garlic powder
1 tablespoon dried chives
1 tablespoon dried parsley
½ teaspoon dried dill
¼ teaspoon kosher salt
⅛ teaspoon freshly ground black pepper

1. In a resealable sandwich bag, combine all the ingredients. Press out the air, seal the bag, and use a rolling pin to lightly crush the chives and parsley.

2. Store in the bag (or in a mason jar) for up to 1 month in the pantry.

ACKNOWLEDGMENTS

Thank you to my partner in cooking and love of yummy food, my brilliant daughter, Sophia. I can't imagine writing books without you helping me. I adore you, my love. Thank you for filling our home with so much affection, love, and laughter.

Scott, thank you for being so honest and kind with recipe testing, and for always doing the dishes when you can tell I'm spent. You've brought so much laughter and joy to my life; thank you for being my safe space.

To my dear friend Heidi and her fantastic family, Ethan, Andy, Pam, and Bruce. Thank you for opening your home and family to me. Thank you for (literally) holding my hand through some of the hardest challenges of my life. I adore you!

To my family, Kara, Joe, Laurie, Alyssa, Aaron, Sean, Lisa, Kaitlyn, Tara, Colin, and Chandler. Thank you for being my band of cheerleaders! I love you all so very much.

To Cindy Epstein, Carl Kravats, and Joni Wilhelm, my wonderful and talented photography team. Working with you is always my favorite part of writing a book. I hope to have many more photo shoots with you in the future!

To my agents, whom I adore, Sarah Passick and Celeste Fine, thank you for helping me realize my dream! Cheers to four books together, and hopefully many more to come!

A special thank-you to all the wonderful people at William Morrow/ HarperCollins for helping me make this book so beautiful and successful! Cassie Jones, Jill Zimmerman, Andrew Gibeley, Heidi Richter, and anyone I've forgotten to mention, this book is a joint effort. I could not have done it without you!

Last, but certainly not least, to my readers. Thank you so much for allowing me into your kitchens. I always try to take all your requests into account (more than 50 percent of this book is vegetarian because of it). Thank you for keeping Lose Weight by Eating a safe space for all, and I urge you to always speak positively about yourself. Self-doubt, body shaming, and speaking negatively about yourself (and others) makes the tough job of weight maintenance that much harder. Next time you look in the mirror, give yourself a compliment. Do this every day for a month, and see how much loving yourself can make your life brighter.

Recipes According to
DIETARY RESTRICTION

EASILY MADE VEGETARIAN

VEGAN

EASILY MADE VEGAN

UNIVERSAL CONVERSION CHART

OVEN TEMPERATURE EQUIVALENTS

250°F = 120°C

275°F = 135°C

300°F = 150°C

325°F = 160°C

350°F = 180°C

375°F = 190°C

400°F = 200°C

425°F = 220°C

450°F = 230°C

475°F = 240°C

500°F = 260°C

MEASUREMENT EQUIVALENTS

Measurements should always be level unless directed otherwise.

⅛ teaspoon = 0.5 mL

¼ teaspoon = 1 mL

½ teaspoon = 2 mL

1 teaspoon = 5 mL

1 tablespoon = 3 teaspoons = ½ fluid ounce = 15 mL

2 tablespoons = ⅛ cup = 1 fluid ounce = 30 mL

4 tablespoons = ¼ cup = 2 fluid ounces = 60 mL

5⅓ tablespoons = ⅓ cup = 3 fluid ounces = 80 mL

8 tablespoons = ½ cup = 4 fluid ounces = 120 mL

10⅔ tablespoons = ⅔ cup = 5 fluid ounces = 160 mL

12 tablespoons = ¾ cup = 6 fluid ounces = 180 mL

16 tablespoons = 1 cup = 8 fluid ounces = 240 mL

INDEX